MEDICAL PRACTICE MANAGEMENT

Body of Knowledge Review
Second Edition

VOLUME 5

Information Management

Medical Group Management Association
102 Inverness Terrace East
Englewood, CO 80112-5306
877.275.6462
mgma.com

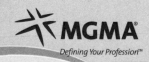

Defining Your Profession™

Medical Group Management Association® (MGMA®) publications are intended to provide current and accurate information and are designed to assist readers in becoming more familiar with the subject matter covered. Such publications are distributed with the understanding that MGMA does not render any legal, accounting, or other professional advice that may be construed as specifically applicable to an individual situation. No representations or warranties are made concerning the application of legal or other principles discussed by the authors to any specific factual situation, nor is any prediction made concerning how any particular judge, government official, or other person will interpret or apply such principles. Specific factual situations should be discussed with professional advisors.

PRODUCTION CREDITS
Publisher: Marilee E. Aust
Composition: Glacier Publishing Services, Inc.
Cover Design: Ian Serff, Serff Creative Group, Inc.

LIBRARY OF CONGRESS CATALOGING-IN-PUBLICATION DATA

Information management.
    p. ; cm. — (Medical practice management body of knowledge review (2nd ed.) ; v. 5)
    Includes bibliographical references and index.
    ISBN 978-1-56829-334-9
1. Medical offices—Management. 2. Medical offices—Automation. 3. Medicine—Practice. 4. Medical informatics. I. Medical Group Management Association. II. Series.
    [DNLM: 1. Information Management—organization & administration. 2. Information Systems—organization & administration. 3. Practice Management, Medical—organization & administration. W 26.55.I4 I4223 2008]
    R728.I44 2008
    610.68—dc22

                                                                      2008044475

Printed in the United States of America
10 9 8 7 6 5 4 3 2 1

Dedication

To our colleagues in the profession
of medical practice management
and to the groups that support us
in our efforts to serve our profession.

Body of Knowledge Review Series — Second Edition

Contents

Preface

INFORMATION MANAGEMENT encompasses the processes and resources required to collect, manipulate, maintain, protect, and retrieve information used in a business enterprise. In health care organizations, as in business and industry, robust information systems and a strong information management capability are acknowledged as strategic resources. As the health care marketplace evolves toward a "seamless" continuum of care, the need for connectivity and sharing of clinical and administrative information among various providers of health services continues to increase. Unfortunately for most organizations, the electronic health record and fully integrated data repositories to support business transactions and patient care activities remain future visions, not current reality.

In their efforts to build and maintain information resources to support clinical and administrative needs, health care executives face numerous challenges, including:

- The speed with which changes in information technology occur;
- Choosing the "right" system from among the plethora of products and services available;
- Facing and addressing the challenge of physician buy-in, and recruiting and retaining their support as key stakeholders;
- Finding and retaining staff with the requisite information skills;

- Increasing information security and confidentiality issues; and

- Ensuring positive cost-benefit perceptions and realities.

In addition to basic foundational knowledge, meeting these challenges (and myriad others inherent in information management) requires a commitment to continued learning, through professional networking and self-directed investigation. The materials in this volume provide this foundational knowledge and guidance for taking the next steps toward maintaining current knowledge in our constantly changing, information-intensive health care environment.

Body of Knowledge Review Series Contributors

Geraldine Amori, PhD, ARM, CPHRM
Douglas G. Anderson, FACMPE
James A. Barnes, MBA
Fred Beck, JD
Jerry D. Callahan Jr., CPA
Anthony J. DiPiazza, CPA
David N. Gans, MSHA, FACMPE
Robert L. Garrie, MPA, RHIA
Edward Gulko, MBA, FACMPE, FACHE, LNHA
Kenneth T. Hertz, CMPE
Steven M. Hudson, CFP, CFS, CRPC
Jerry Lagle, MBA, CPA, FACMPE
Michael Landers
Gary Lewins, FACMPE, CPA, FHFMA
Ken Mace, MA, CMPE
Jeffrey Milburn, MBA, CMPE
Michael A. O'Connell, MHA, FACMPE, CHE
Dawn M. Oetjen, PhD, MHA
Reid M. Oetjen, PhD, MSHSA
Pamela E. Paustian, MSM, RHIA
David Peterson, MBA, FACMPE
Lisa H. Schneck, MSJ
Frederic R. Simmons Jr., CPA
Thomas E. Sisson, CPA
Donna J. Slovensky, PhD, RHIA, FAHIMA
Jerry M. Trimm, PhD, FHIMSS
Stephen L. Wagner, PhD, FACMPE
Lee Ann H. Webster, MA, CPA, FACMPE
Susan Wendling-Aloi, MPA, FACMPE
Warren C. White Jr., FACMPE
Lawrence Wolper, MBA, FACMPE, CMC
Lorraine C. Woods, FACMPE
James R. Wurts, FACMPE

Learning Objectives

AFTER READING THIS VOLUME, the medical practice executive will be able to accomplish the following tasks:

- Develop and maintain appropriate internal communication pathways for clinical and nonclinical staff;

- Develop a technology plan that establishes the criteria for selection and implementation of information technology, including computer systems, Internet strategies, and telecommunications;

- Plan and design a technology security process to protect patient and practice data systems;

- Manage medical information systems, including medical records, medication administration, and health care–related document storage; and

- Develop and implement processes to comply with mandated reports of specified patient issues to regulatory agencies.

1

Vignette # Going Mobile – Is Remote Access Right for Your Practice? [1]

Technology now allows physicians to obtain current patient information easily from home or on the road. Viewing key data such as vital signs and lab results on personal digital assistants (PDAs), cell phones, and "smart phones" is a growing reality at medical groups and hospitals. Remote access to the latest information can be a powerful tool for increasing productivity.

Technical and economic limitations have delayed the application of Wireless Fidelity (Wi-Fi) technologies to clinical information systems and electronic medical records.

■ Wi-fi, Cell Phones Allow Access to Patient Information

Wireless is a broad term – it can cause confusion when people talk about mobile devices operating on various types of networks.

About 70 percent of U.S. hospitals have some type of wireless local-area network,[2] which usually operates within one facility or several buildings of a medical campus. Computer users get online by tapping into Wi-Fi "hotspots." Hospitals and clinics typically use Wi-Fi to transmit clinical information to computers on wheels, laptops, and other medical devices. Clinical information is encrypted, accessible only by authorized users.

In comparison, cellular telephone networks can stretch nation-wide. Most cell phone users can call or text-message from almost any city or state. Smart phones allow users to view Websites, send e-mail and photos, and use office productivity applications.

Wi-Fi networks offer greater bandwidth than cell phone net-works, so data load faster. Yet many places only receive cell phone transmissions. Physicians who are frequently in transit often find a smart phone the best device for obtaining patient information.

◼ Lower Cost, Stark Law Change Make Wireless Devices More Practical

Wi-Fi's price has often prohibited medical groups and rural hospi-tals from using it. However, the cost of the hardware components has dropped significantly.

In addition, in October 2006 the government eased the physi-cian self-referral (Stark) law prohibition on services that hospitals can offer physicians. A medical organization may now provide "reasonable access" to clinical records, including viewing and entering data. One of the main reasons for the change was the gov-ernment's desire to encourage widespread adoption of electronic medical records. This gave medical organizations new options, including the ability to supply physicians with PDAs and smart phones enabling access to clinical information.

◼ Help with Data Gathering, Decision Support

Another factor driving adoption of clinical information systems by provider organizations is the push by Medicare and private payers to collect data for performance measurement. They want the information to improve outcomes and boost patient safety.

Payers sometimes offer provider organizations significant financial incentives to supply desired clinical data sets.

We can expect payers to increasingly deploy clinical decision-support tools for physicians, including patient care plans, electronic prescribing, and diagnostic support tools. They may help reduce medical errors and improve clinical outcomes. Clinical decision-support tools become more effective when linked to real-time patient data, such as vital signs and lab results.

Wireless Challenges

Deploying clinical information systems with wireless accessibility poses challenges for group practice administrators. Who will pay for the devices? What happens if a PDA or smart phone gets lost? What if physicians don't want to use portable devices? However, physicians are already going mobile. A recent report by *Medical Economics* estimated that some 330,000 physicians now use PDAs.[3] The study found that 90 percent of physicians with PDAs use them to look up drug information; about half get some continuing medical education online.

Security of medical information has long been a concern. Laptops can be stolen. Many provider organizations have had the unfortunate task of alerting patients that their medical information has been compromised.

The most advanced clinical information systems are Web based. Data are stored on the provider group's servers. Physicians use Web-based devices to view prescriptions, lab and radiology orders and results, transcribed reports, and other clinical documentation. Data are encrypted and provided in a "view only" mode; they cannot be stored on wireless devices. Thus, if a PDA is lost, it is virtually impossible for an unauthorized person to obtain protected information.

The financial picture is changing, too. Many physicians say financial concerns are the single biggest obstacle to adopting electronic medical records and other new technologies.[4]

In addition to lighter regulatory pressure, clinical information software can be integrated with financial management systems, particularly charge-capture programs. Such software eases work flow, reduces billing errors, and can pay for itself with improved financial performance.

When Motorola introduced the first commercial cellular phone in 1983, it weighed more than a pound and cost $7,000.[5] Over 20 years, technology has made cell phones inexpensive and ubiquitous. In the coming decade we will see similar advances in mobile clinical information.

Current Information Management Issues

INFORMATION TECHNOLOGY (IT), and thus information management, is constantly changing in all industries, not just in health care. In fact, the half-life of some technologies now is counted in months rather than years. Not many years ago, sophisticated information technologies were considered to be prohibitively expensive for all but the largest medical practices, but today the cost of IT is considered an essential business expense. Size still matters, however, and the rate and scope of technology adoption generally is less in smaller practices than in larger ones.

The national agenda for interoperable information technologies distributed across the entire health care system is not new. The potential for IT to "revolutionize" heath care has been widely recognized for many years. Unfortunately, however, the barriers to widespread adoption of integrated IT are real and many. Cost is certainly a prime factor affecting IT adoption, but the complexity of selecting and implementing a technology solution into existing workflow and care processes is an important factor as well.[6]

Under the auspices of the Centers for Medicare and Medicaid Services (CMS) *8th Scope of Work* for the Quality Improvement Organizations (QIOs), IT help may be on the way for medical practices. CMS proposes to make

VistA®, the U.S. Department of Veterans Affairs' electronic health record software, available to physicians for use in their practices. The QIOs, a network of community-based organizations that contract with CMS to monitor the quality of health care for Medicare beneficiaries, will provide free assistance with IT issues to medical practices in their geographic areas. The goal is to aid practices to implement IT as well as to utilize the full functionality of the technology implemented. Physicians involved in the pilot study for this initiative reported positive outcomes related to implementing technology and developing needed skills.[7]

An ongoing Information Management issue that medical practices will deal with for the foreseeable future is compliance with regulations associated with the Health Insurance Portability and Accountability Act of 1996 (HIPAA). HIPAA is one of the most far-reaching pieces of legislation to face health care providers. The "administrative simplifications" are anything but simple – they require medical practices to make numerous changes to their operating processes. HIPAA's Privacy and Security Rules pose challenges as well. Standards for electronic transmission of data include many requirements for which medical practices were not prepared. The full implementation of this legislation will take years, and will continue to make sweeping changes in the business of health care.

Medical practices and other noninpatient health care organizations such as home health have lagged behind the "big players" in the health care system with regard to technology adoption. The reasons mentioned previously (among others) certainly provide rational explanations for this phenomenon. The outcome is that medical practices are now in the unenviable position of needing to make great strides in a short period of time.

Achieving the national goals for systemwide integration of health information and interoperability of IT, as well as meeting the medical practice's unique strategic goals, will require strong leadership from the practice executive. Leadership capability must be supported by a robust knowledge base that encompasses the body of knowledge underlying the medical practice management profession and the Information Management domain.

Perhaps above all else, continued success in managing information resources requires a commitment to continued learning. The rate of change and the volume of change in medical technology fields will only continue to increase. Dependence on technology for managing the delivery of health services will increase concurrently with clinical technology.

Knowledge Needs

THE KNOWLEDGE BASE required to perform information management functions is very broad and draws from several academic disciplines, including management, information systems technology, human relations, and finance. The large body of published literature in this domain incorporates practical reports of actual management experience as well as findings from rigorous research activity.

From a skills perspective, the medical practice executive must be able to perform basic and advanced management tasks, such as those presented in Exhibit 1. Although the skills appear general in nature, they cannot be applied effectively in an information management context without adequate knowledge of the Information Management domain.

Mastering the body of knowledge associated with information management will require delving into the basics of information technology, the current IT market, project planning and management approaches, and education and training methods, among other areas. Academic programs exist that lead to degrees or certification in various aspects of information management (and in health information management specifically). For the medical practice executive, a carefully designed program of self-study is likely an adequate and preferable alternative.

Even though the practice manager may not actually perform all skills and job tasks associated with information management activities in the medical practice, he or she most likely will be responsible for the outcome of those

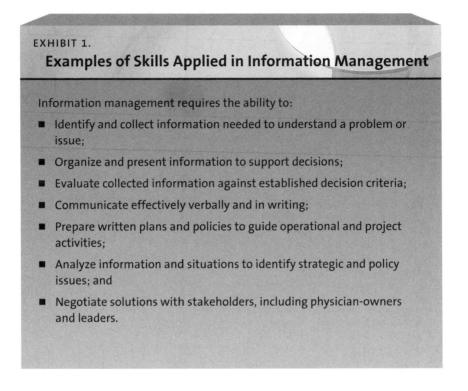

EXHIBIT 1.

Examples of Skills Applied in Information Management

Information management requires the ability to:

- Identify and collect information needed to understand a problem or issue;

- Organize and present information to support decisions;

- Evaluate collected information against established decision criteria;

- Communicate effectively verbally and in writing;

- Prepare written plans and policies to guide operational and project activities;

- Analyze information and situations to identify strategic and policy issues; and

- Negotiate solutions with stakeholders, including physician-owners and leaders.

activities. The practice manager must therefore have a good understanding of the domain tasks and skills to select the right employees for those tasks as well as to evaluate their performance and provide directive feedback. A reasonable level of skill is also required for credibility in professional and leadership roles.

The medical practice executive is ultimately responsible for managing the practice's information resources and accountable for how well those resources meet business and clinical needs. The primary responsibilities include:

- Assessing, understanding, and communicating information resource needs;

- Selecting, negotiating, and securing needed information technologies;

- Managing the implementation of information systems;

- Evaluating staff technical skills and planning for needed training;

- Establishing and maintaining information security practices; and

- Maintaining system viability for maximum utility over the life of the resources.

The degree of expertise in information management skills and knowledge attained is, to some degree, an individual decision based on preference and job requirements; however, a certain level of IT competence is essential.

Chapter 1 **Managing Internal Communication Pathways and Protocols**

◼ Clinical Pathways

Clinical pathways are described as multidisciplinary plans of treatment that are developed to enable the implementation of clinical guidelines and protocols. While best known as clinical pathways, several other terms are used to describe this concept, including care maps, integrated care pathways, and collaborative care pathways. Clinical pathways are utilized to support clinical, resource, and financial management of a patient with a specific condition over a specified time period. The four major components to the clinical pathway include (1) a time line, (2) the type of care, (3) the outcome criteria, and (4) the variance record for identifying deviations from the norms and/or expectations.[8]

The goal of developing and implementing clinical pathways and clinical protocols is to attain a high level of quality of medical care by identifying, implementing, and adhering to specific medical standards by all physicians in a given specialty when treating a specific set of symptoms or identified illness or injury. Through the application of clinical pathways in the utilization of clinical protocols, a group practice will have the tools to generate clinical data that will enable the organization to prove to outside entities the level of clinical quality being provided by the practice.

Clinical pathways and protocols can be derived from multiple sources, including third-party payers, medical specialty societies, and the National Institutes of Health. Even though applying these protocols constitutes good clinical care on its own, the utilization of audits and external assessments to measure compliance with the protocols can be effectively used to confirm the quality of care being provided and therefore justify the negotiation of better contracts with third-party payers and improved relationships with local employers where direct contracting for medical services may be possible.

The effective development and implementation of clinical pathways within an organization requires a multidisciplinary approach, with input from all levels of clinical providers as well as input from nonclinical staff. The initial creation of this type of structure requires the full and unreserved endorsement and support of physicians as well as clinical and executive leadership of the organization. Preliminary meetings and discussions need to be held within the leadership structure to identify the organization-specific goals for the implementation of clinical pathways. In some cases, this may require the inclusion of various community collaborators who have involvement or responsibility for part of the care and treatment plan of the patient. Examples of this outside collaboration may include visiting-nurse services, rehabilitation facilities, and social services support agencies. In addition to being part of the leadership, administrative support goes further in the form of being advocates, facilitators, and champions to show that the organization is in favor of and supportive of the implementation of clinical pathways through both words and the identification and application of necessary financial and operational resources.

In addition, the development and implementation of clinical pathways may have significant effects that go beyond the simple goal of quality care. The development and application of clinical pathway structures, when properly communicated to staff, patients, and community stakeholders, sends a clear and effective message that the practice is committed to maintaining services at no less than industry norms and is effective at both identifying and measuring those norms for improved patient care. Properly designed and implemented clinical pathways will also affect the cost of care through changes in the services that will be rendered based on specific presented symptoms, and may have significant impact on insurance carrier–directed pay-for-performance models. The application of clinical pathways should also increase financial accountability through the elimination of redundancy and variations of clinical methods used by different providers.

In addition to developing and implementing this clinical pathway structure, an organization should create and implement a variety of quality assurance programs to measure the results of the implementation of the clinical pathways and ensure that the desired goals are being reached. The majority of quality assurance programs can be sized to meet the needs of both large and small medical practices. Dependent on the size of the organization, some practices complete their quality assurance programs internally, whereas other practices utilize outside consultants to complete the necessary reviews, audits, and surveys.

A key tool in evaluating adherence to clinical pathways and their effect on the patient population is through the use of various outcomes measures, including chart reviews, whereby a sample of medical records is reviewed to confirm that the proper care is being provided and properly documented in the medical record. Other measurements that can be used include patient and referring-physician satisfaction surveys. These surveys, when completed properly and analyzed in a timely manner, can provide a wealth of information concerning how well the clinical pathways are being received and whether the pathways are in keeping with the standards in the community and the expectations of the patient. The results of these reviews and surveys should be presented to senior clinical and administrative management to enable them to address the issues raised by the results of the surveys and reviews. The data used to define the issues may be perceived differently when reviewed by clinical and administrative staff. Clinicians will be primarily seeking to improve the care being provided to enable the patient to reach the best possible outcome. This goal is important from the administrative point of review as well, but the medical practice administrator is also concerned that the care and service are being provided in the most cost-effective manner with the most efficient use of available resources. Finally, these data are critical to identifying and determining modifications that need to be made in both the strategic and operational planning processes.

◾ Managing Meetings

One of the necessities of organizational governance and operations is the meeting. Meetings are very expensive because they take "billable" time away from the most economically valuable asset of the practice, the physicians. The medical practice executive should consider how much a group meeting will cost in lost productivity and use that as a benchmark to keep meeting times and numbers in check. Meetings are often seen as frequent time wasters, and it is the responsibility of the medical practice executive to recognize this perception and manage it carefully. Meeting management is a practiced art.

For meetings to be effective, they should have many of the following characteristics:

- *A clear task.* Is this an ad hoc or standing group? An ad hoc committee usually performs a specific task and may disband when the task is completed, whereas a standing committee, or a group such as the board, is often covered or mandated in the organization's bylaws. Any meeting body should have a clear expectation of its function and the time line, if necessary, to accomplish its task.

- *Participation.* Members who are selected to attend a meeting, either by appointment or election, should be committed to the group's work and tasks. Absent members can be disruptive because they will need to be brought up to date, and if they disagree with an outcome, work that was thought to be completed may have to be revisited.

- *Expectations.* Expectations should be realistic, and the meeting time should allow participation by all.

- *Rules.* Ground rules for behavior, discussion, and decorum should be established. The meeting should never turn into a hostile situation that might destroy relationships and the past good work of the meeting group. Meetings are rarely good places to resolve personal conflicts and disagreements, which should be taken "off-line."

- *Agenda.* The meetings themselves should have an agenda that is relevant to the governing body or committee meeting. Agendas should not include business related to other governing groups within the practice.

- *Schedule.* The meeting should start and stop on time, as established up front by the time frame indicated on the agenda. The meeting facilitator can show leadership by explaining the reason for hard start and stop times (e.g., respect for everyone's time). One of the greatest failures in managing meetings is an agenda that is too lengthy for the time allowed. The facilitator should assign times for each topic and stick to the times.

A "parking lot" approach will prevent alienating people and potentially losing good ideas. The parking lot is a simple but effective concept that, simply put, acknowledges an idea or topic as valid, but defers it to a future date or to a more appropriate body or person to handle, without taking excessive amounts of meeting time. Depending on the formality of the group, this information can be included in the minutes or simply written on a separate flip chart. The facilitator should follow up with regard to the parking lot issues. If the topic is appropriate for a future meeting, the facilitator should list it on a future agenda. If it is better addressed in another forum, then he or she should direct it there, with feedback to the committee members about the fate of the issue.

Record-Keeping

If careful records of meetings are not kept, several things will happen, none of which are good for the group. Without good minutes, the risk of losing valuable ideas and information about what took place at the meeting is significant. Errors will occur in communication with absent members or in recalling "what happened" at the last meeting. Different versions of the outcomes of many ideas and alternatives will undoubtedly emerge unless a record is kept. Such information, or misinformation, has the potential to spread to others in the group as well. The meeting's minutes are the vehicle for effectively communicating the results of the meeting. If more detail is necessary, an action plan that describes what steps will be taken to complete the activities that were the subject of the meeting is warranted.

Agenda

An example of a meeting agenda is shown below.

Agenda for the Board of Directors
ABC Medical Group
January 1, 2009

1. Call to Order	Chairperson	2 minutes
2. Minutes of the Previous Meeting	Approve	5 minutes
3. Business of the Meeting	Discuss and vote	60 minutes
4. Next Meeting	January 14, 2009	1 minute
5. Adjourn		

The important aspects of this agenda are the specification of the items to be addressed and their allotted times, as well as who is responsible for presenting the topic or what action is needed.

Facilitator

The facilitator, or chairperson, is in charge of the meeting. This means that he or she must keep the meeting on schedule, enforce the rules of decorum and order, use the parking lot approach, and actively seek participation from all members during discussion. The meeting's procedure should be clearly discussed in advance, and agreement needs to be obtained from the participants prior to the meeting.

For meetings to be effective, it is the chairperson's responsibility to watch out for the following adverse actions and to intercede if necessary:

- Personal attacks;
- A member appealing to his or her own expertise or expecting involvement when there is not any reason to do so. This is closely related to the personal attack because it indicts the expertise and work of the members or stakeholders presenting information or ideas and solutions;
- An appeal to popularity (this is very common);
- An appeal for pity (e.g., "poor me");
- A false dilemma, in which only two options to a problem are presented when, in fact, many more are available;
- A complex question for which several answers are required to properly respond, yet because of resource constraints, a variety of answers is rarely presented;
- A false analogy that compares two things that seem to be similar when they are not;
- A slippery slope, which is always very political (e.g., "If we give them a raise, they will expect a raise every year"); or
- An unrepresentative sample, which is a mainstay in rhetoric; a conclusion is drawn (or a decision is made) based on an anecdotal example.

◼ Communicating with the Team

Problem solving and decision making require inquiry. One of the major areas of concern in decision making involves the factors that prevent decisions from being made, sometimes referred to as "decision paralysis" factors. Five paralyses factors are detrimental to the process:

1. Resistance to change (paradigm paralysis);
2. Lack of communication (no collaboration among departments or within some departments);
3. Lack of written guidance (policies and procedures);
4. Lack of employee empowerment; and
5. Lack of recognition of a need to change.

Many organizations fail to recognize the influence of "organizational culture" on the governance process within the entity. Governance flows from culture because the culture of the group will dictate how the group makes decisions.

◼ Communication Plan

For an information management plan to be functional, it will include a structured mechanism for ongoing communication about exposures, policies and procedures, systems improvements, and unanticipated events. Key audiences for information management communication include:

- *The board of directors*, which is ultimately responsible for the safety of patients and corporate compliance;
- *Administration*, which sets the corporate culture's tone;
- *Physicians*, who must understand the corporate expectations and culture within which they are working;
- *Staff*, who take personal risks of retribution when they report an error or potential error and who must understand policies and how to implement them;

- *Patients*, who are called on as partners in today's system to help report inaccuracies on their personal health records; and

- *The public*, who are the practice's constituents.

The communication plan for information management should include both verbal and written communication. Written communication should consider the issue of medical literacy and be written so that laypersons and all staff, including support staff, can understand it. A comprehensive information management communication plan will include:

- *Orientation presentations* for both the board and staff, including the role of information management, the responsibility of the staff and board, and the types of information management involvement expected of them. In addition, the orientation should communicate the philosophy of the organization about the expectation that all staff and the board will participate in ensuring that the organization complies with established standards of safety and corporate compliance.

- *Regular written reports to the administration and board*, including claims, suits, events, near misses, and identified exposures.

- *Regular written communication to staff* to apprise them of exposure and acknowledge them for reporting exposures. Staff are the eyes and ears of the information management process. Unless they are rewarded for exposing information management inefficiencies, deficiencies, and inaccuracies, their participation will be limited. The effective information manager will acknowledge and reward staff participation in information management activities. In addition, staff need to know about actions taken in response to their reports.

- *Corporate communication* through writing for internal newsletters, which should be the responsibility of the information manager whenever possible. The more widely the information management activities are known throughout the organization, the more corporate support is possible.

■ *An understanding of public relations*, especially careful verbal and written communications in situations with high
potential for litigation, for example, those occurring after
an unanticipated event (e.g., a security leak for the electronic health record system). The goal of public relations
is to create a positive image of the organization, and the
information manager must have an understanding of the
implications for liability and legal ramifications. The need
to contain speculations and protect patient confidentiality
while providing sufficient information so as not to be deceptive or perceived as deceptive by the public is paramount.

All staff should be educated about the need to avoid hearsay
and gossip about unanticipated events. Speculation is damaging.
Random musings become facts in the minds of those who share
them. All staff, not just clinical staff, should be trained on the concepts of systems thinking in medical error and the notion of high
reliability as an organizational goal. The more educated staff are in
thinking about safety and the notions of corporate compliance, the
more they can believe the organization is just, fair, transparent, and
striving to improve information and its flow, and the more they will
grasp their role in damage control. Information management can
create plans, processes, and procedures; however, without communication of potential risks and results, there can be no information
management success.

■ Patient Surveys

Patient satisfaction is a time-honored, long-appreciated, but not
often a well-understood factor considered in the improvement of
care. Although patient-satisfaction surveys query specific issues
such as waiting room time, politeness of staff, or even parking convenience, these surveys primarily measure satisfaction with human
interaction. From a patient's perspective, care that is given respect-
fully and communicated well is care that is appreciated and well
perceived.[9] Patient satisfaction measurement tools can provide great
feedback for areas in which improvement in quality of processes can

be applied, and where staff training on communication and interaction with patients and families will improve the overall relationship of the practice to its customers, patients, and families.

Many organizations use standardized surveys, available from vendors such as Press Ganey, which allow for benchmarking against similar practices. Nonetheless, simple tools and phone surveys often yield even more pertinent and effective information. In addition to the traditional and important amenity queries about parking, staff politeness, timeliness, and facility, effective satisfaction surveys will measure perceptions of care appropriateness, thoroughness, and communication. In addition, queries about perception of safety, satisfaction, and patient involvement in decision making are emerging as a result of the increased focus on patient safety and patient-centered care.

The goal of gathering data is to use it to make change. Patient satisfaction data are useless, however, unless they are used. Properly analyzed, such data hold the key to patient retention and reduced likelihood of changing doctors or even litigation. Whatever the methods used by the organization to gather information about patient satisfaction, they should be used to spur change and pinpoint areas for improvement on an ongoing basis.

Data trends should be distributed to appropriate departments and individuals for corrective responses or celebrations of success. Such trends indicate where appropriate quality improvement efforts should be initiated. Customer service training, training in patient-centered care, patient flow processes, or other initiatives can all be monitored through response trends in patient satisfaction surveys. In all cases the data should be communicated with leadership and the board in addition to all staff at least quarterly.

Internal Relations

It is important to maintain effective communications and relations with external customers such as patients, but it is also crucial to communicate with internal customers. Practice executives cannot overlook the importance of their employees and physician-owners.

In other words, if the medical practice executive takes care of the employees, the employees will take care of the patients. Several methods ensure effective communications with employees, including writing a staff newsletter, holding regular staff meetings, establishing an intranet, and providing suggestion boxes.

Staff Newsletter

A staff newsletter can be a vehicle for regular communication with the staff and key stakeholders. Newsletters are an excellent method to reinforce organizational goals and objectives. By using targeted articles, practice executives can include employee success stories that highlight steps in the right direction. The stories not only act as reinforcements, but they also provide employees with recognition.

Another purpose a staff newsletter serves is to provide employees with a periodic update on the current state of affairs. For instance, if part of the practice's goals is to provide on-time service, each newsletter could show the trend toward that goal, along with ideas to help continue a positive trend or new ideas to turn around a negative trend. Another excellent idea is to provide a year-end report to show the practice's final results for each objective. The newsletter can be another method to communicate important information to staff, rather than the traditional meeting or memo.

Staff Meetings

Staff meetings can be an effective way to maintain communication within an organization. These meetings should be viewed as learning opportunities for practice executives and their staff. Meetings can increase the effectiveness and bottom line of both large and small practices; however, if not properly conducted, meetings can waste staff time.

Meetings should therefore have a purpose and a defined agenda. The practice executive should keep the meeting on task; otherwise, participants will lose focus and dread future meetings. Another method to increase the productivity of meetings is to provide staff members with the agenda in advance of the meeting, so they can research the topics for discussion. When staff members are properly prepared, meetings can be effective vehicles for problem solving. One last tip is to follow up all meetings with a thoughtful note to attendees to summarize meeting accomplishments and action plans. This note is more personal than simple meeting minutes sent by e-mail, which typically are deleted without ever being read.

Intranet Communication

An intranet is an internal network belonging to an organization and is typically accessible only by the organization's members. Like the Internet, intranets provide access to information; however, they are secure from unauthorized users and provide organizations with their own personal information resource. Intranet sites can be used to inform stakeholders of what is happening in the practice, changes in practice procedures, upcoming training sessions, continuing-education-unit opportunities, and updates on new governmental regulations. They can also provide links for help.

Suggestion Boxes

Suggestion boxes no longer have to be of the wooden variety. Currently, electronic suggestion boxes are often located on an organization's Website and may also be found on its intranet. The suggestion box located on the external Website, which is accessible via the Internet, can serve to solicit opinions, experiences, and perceptions of customers. Perhaps more important is the suggestion box located within the organization's intranet. Frequently, employees have the knowledge and information necessary to improve the organization; however, they withhold the information for fear of reprisal. This method of communication, if anonymous, can overcome that objection.

Stakeholder Identification and Management

Stakeholders include any individuals or organizations that have an interest in the success of the organization. They can be classified as internal, external, or interface stakeholders. The term *internal stakeholder* refers to any individual who works wholly within the organization, such as office staff. *External stakeholders* refer to individuals and organizations that function outside of the organization, such as vendors, patients, and other physician practices. *Interface stakeholders* are those who function both internally and externally, such as hospital medical staff. Interface stakeholders tend to be quite rare when discussing most types of medical group practices.[10]

Needs/Expectations

The needs and desires of these stakeholders influence the strategy of an organization. Not all stakeholders are equal in terms of their power and influence; in fact, some wield incredible power, whereas others are virtually powerless. Thus, it is necessary to understand the specific demands of each stakeholder so that they can be addressed and satisfied.

Customized Communications

Just like the previously mentioned methods of communicating with internal stakeholders, it is necessary to develop direct communications for external and interface stakeholders. Methods of communicating with this audience include targeted e-mails, direct mailings and newsletters, and conference calls.

Survey Techniques

An effective method of determining customers' needs can be accomplished through the use of survey research. Surveys can also be effective tools to test new ideas or gauge interest in new services as well as to help evaluate a practice's operation. The most common types of surveys are conducted via mail, telephone, or face-to-face – each method having its own advantages and disadvantages.[11]

Mail and E-mail Surveys

Mail surveys are conducted, as the name suggests, via the U.S. Postal Service. Typically, the organization sends surveys to a target audience, and the respondents return them using prepaid, self-addressed envelopes supplied with the surveys. Less expensive surveys can be conducted via e-mail. Inexpensive online resources are available that can assist in the development, collection, and the analysis of results.[12]

The primary advantage of mail and e-mail surveys is the ability to target a large number of respondents with little effort. The major disadvantage is that response rates to mail and e-mail surveys can be quite low. Another potential disadvantage is that respondents may not understand the intent of survey questions and thus may respond inappropriately. This problem is inherent in all surveys and can be minimized by thoroughly pilot-testing the survey to help ensure comprehension.[13]

Telephone Surveys

For a telephone survey, a target audience is selected and contacted by telephone until enough responses have been obtained. The primary advantages of telephone surveys are that they are low in cost and offer the advantage of being able to personally clarify the intention of survey questions. Another advantage is that response rates are typically higher than those received for surface mail or e-mail surveys. Major disadvantages are that telephone surveys are time-intensive and that contact with those on the list is not guaranteed because respondents may not be at home or answer the telephone. Despite the fact that telephone survey response is higher than that for mail surveys, there is usually a high degree of refusal to cooperate.[14]

In-Person Surveys

In-person surveys are conducted face-to-face. An effective method for delivering surveys is to provide patients with surveys during the registration process. A well-designed survey can help patients pass the time until they are called and can help collect valuable information. An advantage of face-to-face surveys, as with telephone surveys, is that the intent of the questions can be clarified. A downside to face-to-face surveys is the perceived lack of anonymity. One solution to this is to have a locked response box for the return of surveys.

■ Culture of Customer Service

A necessary part of interacting with internal and external customers is to project a positive image. One method to achieve this is to instill in your organization a culture of customer service, meaning that all employees should strive to meet and exceed customers' needs, both internally and externally. To do this, medical practice executives need to take the lead and outline expectations; otherwise, the concept of customer service is left open for individual interpretation.

If expectations for delivering customer service and a culture of customer service are not outlined, when a problem surfaces, there is a risk of not only losing a customer, but the practice executive is also faced with reprimanding an employee.[15] These potential issues can be avoided through clear policies and procedures or through initial and ongoing training seminars.

Organizational cultures exist either consciously or subconsciously. Practice executives have the power to choose and shape the culture they want to work within and to transmit that vision to employees and customers. Unfortunately, the culture of customer service doesn't happen overnight, or even in a month. Training can support the change process, but a culture shift requires that internal customers (employees) treat one another with the same dignity and respect that they would award to a guest, and that they trust each other to do the job.[16]

To instill a culture of customer service, practice executives must provide employees with training and the basic tools to deliver customer service. Some topic suggestions include telephone etiquette, cellular phone etiquette, reception desk protocol, dealing with difficult and demanding people, and effective bedside manner.

Telephone Etiquette

Telephones are an essential tool for communication; however, few individuals are versed in their proper use. When answering a business phone, employees should always clearly identify the name of the organization as well as themselves. All too often, employees either forget to do so, or speak so quickly that the name of the organization is unrecognizable. The medical practice executive should develop standard protocols that outline the manner in which phones are answered. Often it is necessary to place callers on hold to deal with patients in person. The protocols should include always asking permission before putting the caller on hold and, after returning to them, thanking them for waiting and completing the conversation. Conversely, when an employee is talking to a patient face-to-face, that conversation should never be interrupted to take a telephone call – that is the purpose of answering machines.[17]

The medical practice executive should emphasize to the staff that when making outgoing phone calls, the key is to respect the caller's time. For example, when making calls to confirm appointments or convey information, staff should always ask whether it is a convenient time to interrupt. Then the caller should deliver the message, answer any questions, and end the conversation.

Cellular Phone Etiquette

Cellular phones are convenient; however, they can invariably interrupt at the most inopportune moments. Policies need to be developed to govern their use in the practice.

Reception Desk Etiquette

"You never get a second chance to make a first impression" is obviously true when a patient encounters the receptionists. Receptionists should always exhibit proper manners. When a person enters the practice, the receptionist should immediately welcome the visitor using a normal tone of voice. All too often, receptionists are either too busy to say "hello," or they tend to "bark out" orders. When possible, receptionists should attempt to use surnames to convey a message of respect to customers. When notifying patients that the "doctor is ready," all efforts should be made to do so in a friendly and calm manner, keeping in mind the patient's ability to react quickly.

Dealing with Difficult People

Often, health care personnel are confronted with difficult people. A primary reason for this is that most patients would rather be somewhere else, and they are anxious about the outcome of their treatment. When encountering individuals who are difficult or defensive, the staff needs to recognize that it is futile to confront such people. They should keep in mind that these persons are insecure and their demeanor is not personal. The staff members should maintain their composure, allow the person to vent, and attempt to provide assistance. One strategy to deal with a difficult person is to empathize with the person and empower him or her by presenting available options to help resolve the matter. If the person becomes abusive, the staff member may consider asking someone else to intercede to deal with the person, or even inviting the person to leave.

Effective Bedside Manner

To deliver customer service excellence, every person in the medical practice must present a caring and genuine manner. This is especially important in the physician/patient relationship. Although physicians are trained to pay attention to patients' emotions and concerns, the realities and time pressures of medical practice make this task difficult. Physicians do not have time to listen to a litany of the patient's psychological complaints, so the strategy often is to "get in there, get the facts, and get out" as soon as possible.[18] Effective bedside manner, however, requires that physicians consider their patients' emotional, social, and family situations. Delivering patient care with a personal touch has tremendous rewards – when patients feel secure and supported, their health is more likely to improve.[19] Physicians need to remember the reasons why they chose health care as a career and to project an attitude of care during every patient encounter.

◾ Summary

Developing community outreach, public relations, and customer relations programs is an essential part of any marketing strategy. It is not necessary for medical practices to engage in all of the strategies presented here to be successful. What is necessary, however, is that the practice executive communicates a well-defined strategy to the staff in order to meet the demands of the community being served.

Chapter 2 **Developing a Technology Plan**

◢ Assessing Information Technology Needs

In years past, medical practice information systems were viewed as necessary for good decision making. Today, effective practice management can occur only when systems are in place not only to provide the information needed for good decision making, but also to assist in performing the actual business and clinical processes. Information management technology is no longer an adjunct, separate "program" that supports the practice; it is a vital, integrated component that will dictate the ultimate success of the practice. Careful assessment of existing capabilities, needs, and potentially advanced systems is required for the development of sustained quality health care provision.[20]

Success comes with efficient processes that eliminate wasted costs, staffing, and energy. But more important in today's environment is the need for systems that ensure outstanding service and clinical quality. Technology can assist in standardizing processes, identifying potential problems, speeding up processes for better outcomes, and improving communications that would otherwise be limited by human capabilities.

The approach to assessing the information technology (IT) needs and then establishing a plan to address those needs is very similar to the overall approach to strategic planning, and in fact should be part of the overall strategy-making process for the organization. This process includes evaluation of existing conditions and systems, consideration of alternatives relative to potential systems, selection of appropriate alternatives, and then implementation of those decisions.[21, 22]

The first step in ensuring that the proper IT is adopted is to understand the processes required in the practice operation and to understand the state-of-the-art technologies available to be integrated into those processes. This analysis usually is undertaken by a team that includes both clinical and business staff, headed by the medical practice executive. Care should be taken to solicit both physician and nonphysician provider input.[23] A clear understanding of the organization's mission, vision, strategy, goals, and objectives is critical to ensuring that the team's efforts will result in a successful implementation.[24]

Evaluating Business Processes

Historically, IT applications to improve medical practice operations were first utilized in business processes. In the current operating environment, most practices handle claims and billing through some type of computerized system. These systems, however, are only a minor part of the overall business processes that can be streamlined, expedited, and standardized to improve the overall quality of the business operations. Every business aspect – from the management of supplies to the disposition of medical waste, from environmental services to utilities and energy management – must be considered to identify potential improvement through the use of available technology.

One of the best methods for identifying and addressing business process needs is to examine the practice's financial statements, considering each line item as a potential location for using technology to improve the bottom line.

Evaluating Clinical Processes

Although every practice has its own unique services, a set of common basic clinical processes can be addressed with a variety of technological systems currently available. Specialty-specific technology that can be added to enhance the basic systems is also available.

The practice manager, in collaboration with the clinicians, should initially identify all the clinical practices that occur. Most of these processes should be known to all, but a good review with the clinicians may turn up specific activities that are handled by the clinicians with little or no communication of their efforts to the staff or practice management.

Cataloging Existing Applications and Tools

Any assessment should start with an inventory of all existing applications. The software may be integrated or may consist of several stand-alone systems. The most common applications are listed in this section. The final inventory prepared by an individual practice should include documentation on each particular software's standard capabilities, the age and costs of existing applications, and – once the applications have been reviewed by the team – their strengths and weaknesses. This information can be entered into a spreadsheet for convenient storage and access for analysis.

Business applications include those that support the operational aspects of the practice, including scheduling, communications, test and data management, and financial transactions. A general listing of common applications follows:

- *Practice management* (e.g., scheduling, reminders, billing, referrals, and authorizations). The heart of an effective system manages the flow of the patient and the information related to the patient: the demographic, financial, and clinical knowledge that is important for moving the patient through the care process. An excellent system will automatically prompt staff as to when and what they need to do, prepare and present the proper information the caregivers need to accurately evaluate and treat their patients, and assist in documenting what was done and accurately bill for the work. Systems also can assist with reminding patients of appointments through automated phone calls and e-mails, thus reducing the number of "no-shows," a major workflow and cost problem for many practices.

- *Services* (e-mail, groupware). More and more providers are choosing to communicate with their patients through e-mail and Internet communications. Additionally, IT is used to coordinate care among caregivers in the practice, practice clinicians, and those who provide referral and specialty care.

- *Claims processing.* Many insurers require claims to be filed electronically. The elimination of the human element in this process reduces errors and speeds the reimbursement in addition to reducing costs.

- *Document processing, spreadsheets, and databases.* Practice management requires various reports and information to adequately understand the business and to report necessary information to stakeholders.

- *Transcription.* Far from the world of basic word processing, today's transcription systems link the physician's thoughts and comments to the electronic health record (EHR); provide key prompts to ensure comprehensive, standard documentation; and allow accurate billing for the services provided. Voice-recognition systems have been slow to develop, but newer systems will include direct dictation.

- *Personnel management.* Staffing is one of the major cost factors for any practice. Accurate records ensure reliable compensation systems and provide management with information to make staffing decisions. For example, with IT, time clocks and manual systems will be replaced by radio frequency identification technology that will detect when employees enter and leave the facility.[25]

- *Inventory management.* As the human element of maintaining inventory is eliminated, carrying costs are reduced and stocking problems and shortages are eliminated.

- *Waste management.* Environmental concerns have pushed waste management programs, which often are elementary in design but have become increasingly crucial to regulatory compliance. Accurate tracking ensures that medical waste is handled properly and helps to document the practice's compliance with all regulations.

- *Energy management.* Recent energy cost increases dictate that facilities control and wisely handle all energy requirements, including electricity, gas, and water usage.

Clinical applications are those that support patient care activities. EHRs are the most widely discussed, but other clinical applications may be distinct for a particular practice. Clinical applications include the following:

- *Electronic health records.* The drive for EHRs originated with the need for easier handling and storage of documentation. Now EHRs are critical support tools for ensuring quality care and for enabling accurate billing for services.

- *Prescription management.* Newer prescription systems allow good documentation for care, guard against conflicting medications, and allow proper oversight for detecting misuse and abuse.

- *Disease management.* Proactive disease management programs allow the provider to assist the patient in undertaking interventions rather than waiting until reactionary efforts are required. Relatively new on the scene, disease management systems are expected to reduce the overall costs of care for chronic diseases and allow a higher quality of life for those affected.

Patient applications are emerging as crucial marketing and service delivery methods in medical practices. Some of the more common applications currently employed include the following:

- *Electronic communication* (Website, e-mail). As an increasing number of patients take the initiative to explore their health problems and actively participate in their own care, physicians must be able to provide accurate and timely information. Many medical practices establish Websites and other programs so patients can communicate with the provider electronically. Done properly and with adequate security, these programs can speed care delivery and recovery. For example, such applications can facilitate speedy prescription refills, make appointments, and report follow-up information to the provider without the effort and cost of an office visit.

- *Electronic monitoring.* Telephone lines and the Internet allow many patients with chronic conditions to regularly report and monitor their physical conditions. This is especially beneficial to those who are unable to drive or travel. Continuous monitoring of body temperature, blood pressure, and heart rates can allow the provider to be alerted instantly when the patient experiences a problem. Implanted defibrillators, a common health maintenance item, can now be monitored through wireless Internet connections for faster response by caregivers and clinical providers.

- *Education via Internet.* In addition to providing information that can assist patients with their own management of health problems, the Internet offers opportunities for encouraging the patients to participate in wellness and health promotion activities.

- *Telehealth.* Although the days of physician visits to the home may be all but gone, through the Internet and telehealth programs, clinicians may be able to conduct patient examinations without the need to travel. Two-way links between the provider's offices and the patient's home or business may allow for quick and effective consultations that reduce the cost of travel and time away from the home or office.

Inventory of Existing Hardware

Once the software and applications have been determined, the hardware that supports the systems should be identified. In addition to specifying what equipment is in place, the connectivity of the equipment needs to be specified. Some equipment may be capable of supporting or connecting with other systems, whereas some may be strictly independent. Overall strengths and weaknesses of the equipment should be identified. The evaluation of the hardware and its flexibility will provide a basis for the long-term planning for support of the systems.

Workstations are the interface points between humans (e.g., care providers and support personnel) and the IT systems that assist in providing quality care to the patients. These data entry and retrieval points have evolved from simple hardware components, formerly placed in the back rooms of the office area, to mobile information centers that connect with real-time information at the point-of-care. Early workstation versions usually consisted of personal computers (PCs) or components that performed transaction-processing activities to provide data and information for patient care and billing. Today, the workstation is more likely a tablet PC or a personal digital assistant (PDA) that the provider uses in place of paper documents. As a result of these innovations, data access and documentation time has decreased, and the provider has more time to spend directly with the patient. Direct data entry improves the quality of documentation, provides more accurate billing, and increases patient satisfaction.

Servers are hardware components, similar to those in normal PCs, that provide the "brains" of the information systems. Servers have replaced large mainframe computer hardware because of their flexibility and robust capabilities. The equipment usually is developed for 24-7 operation. Therefore, servers are more durable than regular PCs and actually may contain redundant components providing backup to ensure continuous stability of service. Multiple servers can be connected to enhance capacity and service. Servers have recently been constructed in high-density modules known as "blade" servers that can provide powerful systems in small spaces. Blade servers are intended for use with single dedicated applications, such as Web pages.

As mentioned, many new practice management systems have replaced large stationary workstations with *handheld devices* that allow point-of-service entry of information. Most of these come in the form of tablet PCs or PDAs. These devices are small enough to be carried into the exam room and used by the provider while interacting with the patient. Often, the device is wirelessly connected to the main information system so data are captured in real time. Records and files maintained on servers and in central storage devices are automatically updated. These systems usually provide boiler-plate information templates and touch-pad entries for faster data capture. A template can capture and store a larger volume of information than a free-text format. Ideally, data input at the time care is given will result in improved quality of information and better subsequent care.

In addition to using PDAs and tablet PCs, medical staff can collect information directly from *monitoring devices*, which completely eliminate the transfer of data. Examples of some of these include monitors for IV pumps, blood pressure, temperature, and heart rate.[26]

Portals allow authorized users to gain entry to information systems. Access can be granted to patients so they can easily find pertinent information about their health and the care provided by the medical practice in a "one-stop" environment. Patients can access health record information, health educational materials, care instructions, clinical data, pharmacy and drug information, and billing information. Portals can also provide access to providers via secure e-mail and facilitate online appointment making.

Captured data may be stored on in-house PCs or on a centralized server, either on site in the facility or in an off-site data bank. Outsourcing data storage is often used to ensure data security. As the cost of electronic storage (e.g., CDs and DVDs) has decreased, it has become the preferred medium compared to hard-copy systems because of its speed and ease of access.

▉ Data Security

The importance of data security transcends all aspects of the software and hardware components of information management systems. A review of the systems with respect to the security of the information, whether financial, clinical, demographic, or personal, should be made while inventorying the resources of the systems. The three-fold approach established by the Health Insurance Portability and

Accountability Act (HIPAA) is an excellent method for reviewing the systems.[27]

The first review in the HIPAA approach should be of administrative systems, including the backup systems, disaster recovery systems, and emergency-mode operational capabilities. The second level of review should be of physical resources. This will include both hardware and software for workstations and storage media, as well as the overall physical facility. Finally, the technical aspects of the systems should be reviewed, including the authentication and transmission of data programs, data integrity systems, and other control systems.[28]

◼ Strategic Information Partners

The information needs of the medical practice are not the only reasons for performing an IT assessment. The needs of organizations and entities with which the practice interacts should be considered as well. For example, organizations that process payment for health care and those that provide adjunct support services, such as reference laboratories, diagnostic facilities, and hospitals to which patients are referred, all have information needs. Planning for providing the information these entities require in an efficient, seamless process strengthens working relationships and reduces costs for all parties involved.

Insurance companies, Medicare, Medicaid, TRICARE, and other third-party payers collect increasingly more data on their customers. Through data analysis, they hope to provide interventions that improve their beneficiaries' health, and thus lower costs of care overall. Information from medical practice records is useful to track patients' compliance with interventions. Data-mining programs can provide better information regarding the efficacy of treatments.

Because policy interest is placed on the quality of outcomes, the costs of specific treatment programs, and disease management, regulatory agencies monitor activities and treatments more aggressively. The monitors search for better outcomes associated with a given approach and watch for abuses and misuses that may be occurring.

Reference labs and diagnostic centers used by medical practices require clinical and financial information that practices typically collect. It is important to find ways to share this information in a confidential manner. Shared information can yield cost and quality improvements for both the medical practice and the diagnostic service.

Inpatient programs need to know the treatments and drugs the medical practice has provided to a patient prior to admission. The availability of current clinical information prevents duplication or omission of needed care and facilitates timely response to patient needs. In addition, the patient's financial information is required to facilitate the reimbursement process.

■ Gap Analysis

Physicians, nonphysician providers, and practice staff often feel frustrated with existing systems, especially if these systems are older and inefficient or are not integrated. Perhaps the existing systems don't fit the current workflow or the personal "rhythm" of a physician's process for working up and caring for patients. Stopping the clinical thought process or interrupting it while making entries into an information system may result in lost time, mental fatigue, and at times create a situation in which quality is compromised. Or it may be that the existing system may not provide the appropriate information for the practice or its strategic partners. In both these cases, clear gaps exist between what is needed and what is available. Finding a solution requires not only an understanding of the problem, but also knowledge of the technologies and systems available to fix the problem. Gap analysis should identify areas of dissatisfaction with existing systems, needs for planned business process changes, needs for planned clinical service changes, and any desired patient applications.

A survey of the clinicians and other practice staff will determine whether existing systems satisfy their job needs to their levels of satisfaction. Be aware that clinicians may not be immediately cognizant of problems or opportunities for improvement because of their experience and comfort with the existing system, which may have led to their acceptance of an existing, inefficient process.

Changes in reimbursement filing requirements or additional regulatory reporting may dictate necessary modifications in processes. These changes should be considered during the evaluation with regard to system needs for the revised processes. Any new or modified services should be documented, and special note should be made of the required information and processes resulting from these changes.

Communications with patients traditionally have been person-to-person, but many patients prefer (and sometimes insist) that their contact with a clinician be through electronic media. The practice must assess whether its patient base is sophisticated enough for the practice to offer the Internet, e-mails, and Websites as standard communication modes. Some practices may prefer to keep in contact using "e-zines," electronic magazines or newsletters by which the physicians can pass on the most up-to-date research and information about health and wellness.

In addition to the dissemination of information, both private and communal, the practice may also need to consider telehealth programs that allow the patient to provide the practice with ongoing data such as blood pressure, glucose levels, and other metrics that can be transmitted over telephone lines or the Internet.

◼ Planning Future IT Architecture

One of the most difficult aspects of technology planning is predicting the future. Technology changes quickly, and seldom in a linear fashion. Tremendous amounts of time can be expended attempting to monitor and assess the state of the art within the industry. Often this is an area for which the practice may wish to employ outside assistance.

The practice should consider its strategic plan and the overall mission and vision of the organization. If the practice is considering growing or changing services, or becoming part of a larger or different organization, its future IT requirements may be dramatically different from those for the current clinical practice.

For the medical practice executive, monitoring trends is a time-consuming but necessary requirement for determining the proper direction for moving the IT program. Again, this is an area where outside assistance from an expert consultant may be valuable. A plethora of journals exist that can provide insight into current trends and their likely future directions. Reliable IT vendors are a key source of information, not only about their own systems but about industry trends as well. Support agencies such as the Medical Group Management Association provide seminars, books, and other materials that can help.

The desired long-term IT commitment may vary due to the overall culture of the organization. The organization's place in the local health care community should be considered, along with the desire or need to compete with other local medical practices or alternate care sites. The emphasis on IT will vary, based on what others are doing and the executive and strategic goals for the organization. More sophisticated IT programs require more oversight and guidance. The level of emphasis and support provided by the management of the organization can affect the decision about which systems to select.

Although new information systems require less space than earlier systems because of their more compact design, the physical space requirements should still be considered. Proper ventilation, security, and utility support may dictate limits to hardware selections. Off-site or outsourced services may be required.

The lack of existing staff with the necessary IT support skills, or an inability to recruit such staff, may result in a decision to outsource IT services. A clear understanding of the system requirements for maintenance and upkeep of the system should be made before selecting the equipment. If the practice staff is not capable of supporting the new systems, serious problems could result. The costs for providing long-term internal support vs. the costs for outsourcing should be carefully compared.

Initial capital investment cost is often the least-expensive component of an IT decision. Typically, the first year of operational support is built into the purchase agreement, but subsequent costs for upkeep may negate any initial benefits. Ongoing costs for staffing/consultation, support, updates, and hardware maintenance can overwhelm a medical practice, particularly a smaller one. Serious consideration must be made of the overall costs for the IT investment over an extended time. A five-year projection of costs and return on investment will provide insight into the true value of the system.

◼ Planning for Implementation and Process Changes

Standard planning, decision-making, and project management tools can be used to evaluate and determine the proper components of the new IT program. These tools can be broken down into three different areas, as summarized in Exhibit 2.

The first group, initial planning tools, will assist in organizing and initiating the process. Team design and development methods taken from standard total-quality management systems will get the process started. Basic communications systems for the team should be established. A strategic management review should be undertaken early in the process, including reviewing the mission, vision, goals, and objectives.

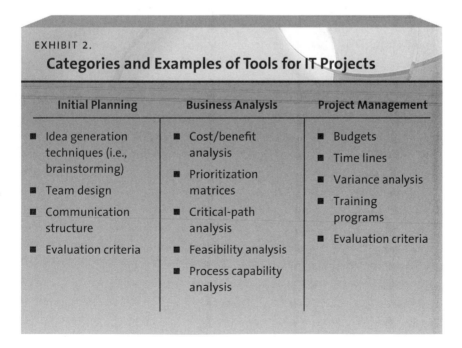

EXHIBIT 2.

Categories and Examples of Tools for IT Projects

Initial Planning	Business Analysis	Project Management
▪ Idea generation techniques (i.e., brainstorming) ▪ Team design ▪ Communication structure ▪ Evaluation criteria	▪ Cost/benefit analysis ▪ Prioritization matrices ▪ Critical-path analysis ▪ Feasibility analysis ▪ Process capability analysis	▪ Budgets ▪ Time lines ▪ Variance analysis ▪ Training programs ▪ Evaluation criteria

The second group, business analysis tools, should be employed once fundamental information is collected. These tools should include cost/benefit analysis, systems prioritization, and critical-path analysis for implementation time frames.

Finally, project management systems will help with the actual implementation once the key systems decisions are made. The team should agree on metrics that will assess the success of the implementation and the ultimate success of the IT programs.

For a good review of classic management and planning tools, go to www.skymark.com/resources/ and select Classic Tools from the Management Resources pull-down menu. Some vendor sites include lists or links to tools used specifically in IT management. One example is available by choosing the Books and Tools selection at www.mde.net/cio.

◼ Assessing Readiness for Change

Resistance to change is an ever-present problem when planning modifications to IT systems. Staff and clinicians alike have usually become comfortable with existing systems. They may worry about the time and energy required to learn new systems and processes, despite their awareness of the potential for improved efficiency and outcomes. Informal discussions with staff can provide insight into the existence or extent of their "change anxiety." Resistance should be met with open, clear communications about the planned changes. The level and intensity of these communications should be determined by the level of resistance encountered.

Before the process is started, everyone should understand the personnel requirements necessary to plan and implement the changes. The staff and clinicians affected by the changes should understand the required efforts and tasks and should be comfortable about their capabilities to perform those requirements. If there is a void in the capabilities of the existing staff, outside consultants or support may be necessary.

Chapter 3 **Facilitating Information System Procurement and Installation**

◾ Selecting an Information Technology Solution

Because selecting and purchasing an IT solution is a major decision, it should unquestionably be based on careful planning and evaluation. The first step is to identify a relatively large group of potential vendors who offer the applications or services the practice is seeking to acquire. Information typically will be gathered from a variety of sources, including print and online media, direct sales marketing, and personal recommendations.

◾ Establishing a Selection Committee

The selection and final decision for purchasing an IT solution should not be made by one individual, not even if that person is the medical practice executive. Instead, the selection should be made by a committee comprised of end users of various aspects of the proposed system, the medical practice executive, physician leaders, and representative staff. This selection committee will assist with the following aspects of the selection process:

- Identifying vendors;
- Categorizing vendors;

- Developing the *request for information (RFI)*;
- Assessing RFI responses;
- Developing the comparison matrix;
- Developing the *request for proposal (RFP)*;
- Assessing RFP responses;
- Collecting information from references;
- Making site visits to vendor clients; and
- Selecting the finalist.

Evaluating Vendor Proposals

One major source for identifying vendors offering potentially useful information management products is through trade shows. Visiting as many vendors as possible in an exhibit situation allows for rapid gathering of information and quick comparisons of major product attributes. If the trade show is in conjunction with a professional association meeting, it is possible to network with colleagues for recommendations, especially if they are seeking similar products or have already implemented similar technology solutions.

Additional sources of information about products to investigate and consider for purchase include trade publications (printed or on the Web), promotional materials received through direct marketing, and resources provided through Medical Group Management Association® forums.

Once an acceptable number of prospective vendors has been identified, the list will require some preliminary manipulation and refinement to become a useful tool to guide the investigation. Categorizing the vendors in a logical framework will facilitate comparison on key variables. Categories may include portal type, market niche served, specific functionality requirements, or some other grouping that is meaningful to the practice. Sorting the vendors into categories helps target those offering key products and services under consideration and shows where more information about their products and services is needed. This process may eliminate some vendors for various reasons.

The vendors remaining on this initial list should be sent an RFI. The RFI collects a standard set of information on each vendor to enable comparison on similar products. Amatayakul[29] recommends a two- or three-page set of questions in the following areas:

- *Company background* – information on the vendor's size and financial stability;

- *Product information* – product name, primary market, technical platform, and overview of product capabilities (later, this will be matched with key functionality criteria);

- *Market information* – vendor identification of its major competitors and explanation of how it differs from the competitors;

- *Installed base and clients* – number of product sales, number of projects in implementation, and number of full installations; and

- *Special criteria* – unique features or functions desired by the practice.

As responses to the RFI are received, an information base will help to analyze the vendors on important company characteristics and product functionality. A commonly employed method is to create a comparison matrix, which can be easily constructed in a spreadsheet application such as Microsoft® *Excel*. Such a matrix allows easy visual comparison of the data obtained, and the spreadsheet works well to apply a ranking scheme. Thorough review of the data supplied in response to the RFI and analysis of the extracted data in the comparison matrix helps to narrow the number of vendors to a "short list." The Better Business Bureau can supply information on any complaints filed concerning particular vendors.

The committee will now seriously investigate the vendors on the short list. More, and more-detailed, information will be required to make a final choice. The next step is to submit an RFP to the short-list vendors. The RFP will specify all the system requirements defined by the practice and solicit a detailed, official proposal from each vendor. The format and content of an RFP will vary across organizations, but most RFPs and vendor proposals will include the information categories shown in Exhibit 3.

EXHIBIT 3.

RFP and Vendor Proposal Content

Category	Request for Proposal	Expected Proposal Content
Selection Criteria	This section should explain to potential vendors the criteria that will be used in the practice's evaluation process.	The vendor should know and acknowledge the most important elements affecting the purchase decision and how the various rating criteria will be weighted.
Practice Profile	The RFP should contain a description of the practice, including its basic demographics, mission, and goals, organizational structure, services provided, and current information infrastructure. In addition, activity information, such as number of patients seen per day, number of modalities performed, number of employees, number of physicians, and number of departments expected to use the application, may also be provided.	This information helps the vendor understand the purpose, size, and complexity of the practice as well as the type of activity and volume of transactions the application will be expected to handle. The vendor's response should address these capabilities.
Specific Platform	The RFP must specify the functional and technical requirements for the proposed system. Any specific features or functionality must be described.	The vendor's response should indicate whether its product currently has the listed function/feature or whether the feature is planned for development. The vendor should describe the technical environment (hardware, network, software) required for its application to operate effectively and efficiently.
Price Range	The RFP should request quotes of one-time cost estimates as well as recurring costs for system maintenance.	The vendor's response should provide the cost of implementing its proposed technology solution to meet the specified functional and technical requirements.
Delivery Time Line	The RFP should describe the vendor's expected deliverables and state the practice's desired time line for various aspects of project implementation and completion.	The vendor should respond with specific, accurate feedback about its ability to comply with the time line.

continued on next page

EXHIBIT 3. *(Continued)*
RFP and Vendor Proposal Content

Category	Request for Proposal	Expected Proposal Content
Ongoing Service	The RFP should outline the practice's system maintenance expectations.	The vendor's response should describe maintenance plans and options available to the organization.
References/ Portfolio	The RFP should request a list of references from other clients similar to the practice in size and type, and clients that implemented the products under consideration.	The vendor should provide a list of clients that may be contacted for interviews and on-site demonstrations of the implemented product.
Other Criteria	The practice should require the vendor to outline training and support policies and procedures.	The vendor may have specific training and support plans that apply to its products. All training and support should be mapped out, as well as any additional training and support that may need to be purchased separately.

As responses are received, the medical practice executive should review the proposals, again using a comparison matrix, and identify the most qualified vendors. The executive should take this opportunity to "sell" or report back to physician leadership. The physicians are often the owners of a medical practice and any venture into a new system should be portrayed in a positive light – as an "investment."

As qualified vendors are identified, the selection committee should contact the references listed by the vendor. In addition to discussing general pros and cons of the application and the vendor, the following factors should be discussed with reference clients:

- Overall quality and reliability of the product;
- Product performance under operating conditions;
- Quality of after-sale service and support;
- Trustworthiness of vendor and its sales representatives;

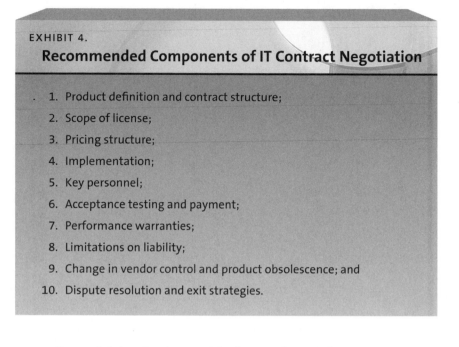

EXHIBIT 4.

Recommended Components of IT Contract Negotiation

1. Product definition and contract structure;
2. Scope of license;
3. Pricing structure;
4. Implementation;
5. Key personnel;
6. Acceptance testing and payment;
7. Performance warranties;
8. Limitations on liability;
9. Change in vendor control and product obsolescence; and
10. Dispute resolution and exit strategies.

- Ease of doing business with the vendor; and
- Openness of future strategies and plans.

The complexity of the RFP responses may make evaluation impossible without a visit to a client site where the application is actually being used. The site visit, in addition to being an opportunity to discuss the pros and cons of the application and the other issues identified above, also becomes a perfect opportunity to view a live demonstration of the application.

Just as with the RFI, creating a spreadsheet matrix of all items in the RFP as well as information gathered from references can greatly assist with the final evaluation and selection. A rating or ranking scheme should be applied to the selection factors, with system functionality, overall quality of the technology, sale and maintenance price, and customer support services typically given higher weights. After a weight has been established for each criterion, the selection committee should rate each vendor on all criteria. When the individual scores are added, the vendor with the highest total points typically is chosen for contract negotiations. Sometimes "make-or-break" factors are identified early in the process to eliminate vendors that cannot provide an essential service.

Negotiating Vendor Contracts

Contract negotiation begins with incorporating content from the RFP and the vendor's proposal into the vendor's standard contract template. The contract should clearly define performance expectations and include penalties if requirements are not met. The medical practice executive should give special attention to the schedule, budget, responsibility for system support, support response times, and upgrades. The practice manager should ensure that all payments to the vendor are tied to completion of milestones and acceptance of deliverables. The Healthcare Financial Management Association has compiled a guide to IT contract negotiation that identifies the 10 critical components shown in Exhibit 4.[30]

Chapter 4 **Developing and Implementing Information System Training and Support Programs**

◢ Implementing Training and Support Programs

One of the most important factors In creating any type of training or employee development program is to determine explicitly what training needs to be given. This premise is as important in designing training programs for information systems applications as it is for other skill-based activities in the medical practice. Early in the planning process, the practice manager should establish the expected learning outcomes, that is, the knowledge and skills that are expected to exist at the conclusion of the training. As an immediate follow-up, the manager should determine the staff's existing knowledge and skill levels. Simplistically, the "gap" between what is already known and what should be known determines the content of the training program. Realistically, though, not all individuals will be at the same beginning skill level, and not all individuals will achieve the same outcome skill level. Therein lies the challenge – how to design (or purchase) effective training programs that meet the diverse needs of the staff and are also efficient and cost-effective from a business standpoint.

The key is to establish evaluation criteria based on recognized characteristics of "good" training and education programs. These criteria can be used to evaluate purchased training services or to serve as guidelines for developing in-house efforts. In general, good training programs are:

- Designed with clearly established and clearly communicated outcome goals;

- Delivered in an efficient manner that draws from and builds on the staff's existing knowledge; and

- Structured to develop knowledge and skills that have immediate utility for the learner.

Assessing Staff Training Needs

The manager should consider several factors in planning training for a new system implementation or system upgrade. Business staff and clinical staff in the practice will use different aspects of the information system's functionality; therefore, training needs will need to be assessed separately for each group.

One way to collect data about the staff's current knowledge and preferences for training programs is to survey them. Based on staff size and the amount of information needed, the survey may be as formal as a written document to be completed and returned to the medical practice executive, or as informal as an e-mail message with a few questions sent to all staff members.

Selecting Training Approaches

Any type of learning is achieved primarily through five generic approaches: reading, hearing, seeing, saying, and doing. Training activities that use more than one of these methods will produce better learning and retention than single-method approaches. By far, however, people learn more by *doing*. Exercises in which staff practice the new skills and apply what they are learning in different situations is key to effective learning.

Characteristics of Adult Learners

It is important to consider personal characteristics associated with working adults related to training preferences. For example, most adults prefer *task- or problem-centered* training. This means that the more a learning activity simulates a real problem encountered in a job, the more likely the staff will learn the underlying facts or concepts associated with a correct action or solution. Working adults also tend to be more enthusiastic about training and education that is relevant to their current job tasks. Another characteristic typical of working adults is that they generally are very pragmatic, which may be demonstrated as a preference for "just in time" and "just enough" learning. They are more likely to use new skills on their job immediately after training is completed.[31]

The "learn by doing" principle is applied in most on-the-job training for staff development by using one of four broad categories of approaches:

- Lecture and/or demonstration to a group;
- Self-learning with print materials;
- Technology-assisted learning; or
- One-on-one training with a facilitator.

Each approach is useful for specific purposes, and each has advantages and disadvantages. A good, basic discussion of these types of training approaches and evaluation criteria for selecting the most appropriate one for a given situation is presented by Mygrant and McMann.[32] Selecting the teaching method or methods to use for training in information management applications will likely be based on such factors as:

- Desired learning outcomes;
- Complexity of content or skills to be learned;
- Number of individuals to be trained;
- Length of time available for training; and
- Training budget.

Train All or Train-the-Trainer

Among the first questions the medical practice executive should consider are whether all staff will need to be trained and whether they will require the same training. More likely, training needs will differ by job position. Specifically, who in the organization needs to be trained and how do their training needs differ?

In some instances, it may be best to select one or a few individuals who can learn the required skills relatively quickly because of their existing knowledge base or aptitude for information management technology. These individuals may receive broad-based training (from the vendor or through self-instruction) and then provide more personalized instruction to practice staff who need skill only in a specific system functionality. This "train-the-trainer" approach can be an efficient and cost-effective way to provide differing levels of instruction to staff with diverse job requirements related to the information system and its various applications. Some staff may be more comfortable learning from co-workers than from professional trainers. This approach is particularly suitable for those who prefer just-in-time and just-enough training.

On-Site vs. Off-Site Training

A final factor to consider in selecting the training approach is to determine whether training should occur on site or off site. As with other factors, each option has merits and drawbacks. Although the key points to consider are relatively simple, the answers may not lead to a clear decision. The final choice may require some accommodations to minimize uncontrollable negative factors. These key points are:

- Whether training on site will disrupt practice operations;
- Whether staff will have adequate job downtime to concentrate on training as needed;
- Whether staff can be relieved of job duties to go off site;
- How important it is for staff to apply the training in the operating environment to maximize its utility; and
- Whether training on the new system can occur concurrently with implementation.

■ Time Analysis

The medical practice executive should determine the time required to complete training for all affected staff as realistically as possible. Creating a work schedule that maximizes staff productivity can be a daunting challenge in itself. Establishing a training schedule that doesn't adversely affect the work schedule can be even more so. Nevertheless, it is important that all staff who are expected to use the information system receive training to use it correctly and efficiently. Inadequate training can result in work process inefficiency and costly (and sometimes dangerous) errors, as well as staff frustration and dissatisfaction. Staff may perceive the system as too difficult and seek ways to avoid using it.

The medical practice executive should establish a schedule that provides training first to staff members in key positions – those individuals whose use of the information system is critical to business and clinical operations. Adequate time should be allowed to ensure that key staff master the required skills before moving on to train the next level of information system users. The schedule also should include makeup options – if training occurs on site during operating hours, the demands of the work environment may require staff to abort training sessions to deal with pressing business or clinical matters. Retraining needs should be considered as well. Few people can master difficult skills or change existing procedures in one session. It is usually a good plan to provide instruction, spend some time using the application, and return to the training mode to respond to questions or to verify that learning has been sufficient.

■ Cost Analysis

The training budget is an important element of the overall cost/benefit analysis for system implementation. The medical practice executive should investigate several cost factors for the analysis. Key factors include trainer costs, personnel costs, equipment and training materials, and various miscellaneous (usually hidden) costs.

Training by vendor personnel may be included in the purchase price of the information system or it may be an "add-on" option that is priced separately. The medical practice executive, who may be very familiar with the system through the selection process, may underestimate the amount of training that will be required for staff with no previous orientation to the system. In some cases, the training price may seem "high" relative to the expected amount of training required, and the practice manager may misjudge the cost/benefit of training to the bottom-line value of the system.

The medical practice executive should realistically evaluate the cost of purchasing training against the difficulty staff may have in migrating to the new application(s) without training, as well as the effect a long self-learning curve may have on system implementation. A system that cannot be used efficiently or that requires a long phase-in period while staff learn its functionality may be more costly than the price of training.

Employees should be compensated directly for the time spent in training. Lost productive time while staff are in the training sessions, however, is often an unforeseen – and sometimes surprisingly large – cost. As noted previously, the productivity issue may be a consideration in deciding when and where training will occur. In some cases, such as a limited system upgrade, staff may be trained effectively while continuing to do their daily jobs. In other cases, staff should not reasonably be expected to work and train concurrently; one or both of the expected outcomes – production or learning – will be less than satisfactory.

Unless all training equipment is provided by the trainer, those costs should be determined as specifically as possible. Room rentals and projection equipment can add several hundred dollars per day of training to the budget. The medical practice executive must understand how costs are affected by where training occurs and the practice's responsibility for bearing those costs.

Although training materials generally are prepared by the trainer, and the cost of the materials usually is included in the training fee, the medical practice executive should question whether all materials will be provided and in what format. For example, help manuals and other learning resources provided electronically may need reproduction into a hard copy for efficient use, which can add significant hidden costs.

Miscellaneous costs are more difficult to anticipate and quantify. Talking with colleagues who have been "burned" by unplanned costs may be the most useful source for this type of information. In the final analysis, some costs will remain unknown and perhaps unknowable. Each budgeting process can be a learning experience to inform the next process.

Evaluation of Instruction and Learning

Evaluating the effectiveness of training programs is generally the responsibility of the medical practice executive. Unfortunately, this crucial task often goes undone; some authors estimate that fewer than 10 percent of staff education programs are evaluated adequately.[33]

The medical practice executive should establish the criteria for evaluating the training programs in the early stages of planning the program. In general, these should include outcome measures for effectiveness, efficiency, and cost. When considered in the aggregate, these measures will help in assessing the value of the training program to the practice.

Regarding effectiveness, the primary focus is whether the desired learning occurred – do staff members now have the desired knowledge and skills initially established as outcome goals for the training program? This measure can examine staff in the aggregate or look at individuals. Broad measures include whether all staff received the training and whether all staff demonstrated a minimum level of proficiency. However, it may be more useful to examine individual learning outcomes as part of the overall staff performance evaluation process.

Efficiency measures determine whether the learning occurred with expenditure of reasonable or acceptable resources, primarily considering resources associated with time and operational impact. For example: Was the training period within the estimated time line? How many worker hours were allocated to training? What was the overall effect on productive staff time? Was operating revenue lost because of training time? Were projections appropriate, or were variances significant?

Although the total actual cost of the training certainly is important, the focus should be on assessing actual costs relative to budgeted costs. The choices of training options were based in part on the expected cost of those options, but would those same choices have been made if the true costs had been known? Each budget variance should be investigated to determine the underlying cause. Was the variance due to cost items not anticipated and planned for? Was the variance due to errors in estimation within cost categories? Cost analysis should be viewed as a learning process rather than a punitive exercise. Again, knowledge gained through this analytical process informs the choices made in future processes.

■ Providing Access to Electronic Education and Information Resources and Systems

Today's health care work force has access to more opportunities for professional development and continuing education than can be cataloged. High-quality programs are available on almost any topic of interest, and many programs are available in electronic formats that can be accessed at the workers' convenience. The savvy medical practice executive will determine which technology-based training solutions will provide the greatest value to clinicians, to operating staff, and, in the long run, to the practice.

■ Resource Options

Available education resources are numerous, have a wide range of costs (both financial and in terms of worker time), and are highly variable in their utility and quality. Managers planning for the education and professional development needs of the practice likely will draw from a variety of sources, but they may rely primarily on a few "tried and true" known sponsors. Representative categories of education sponsors include professional associations, proprietary organizations, and academic institutions. Perhaps most well-known to the medical practice executive is the Medical Group Management Association (MGMA).

MGMA Knowledge Base

MGMA offers a large volume of educational and practice resources of benefit to practice managers, clinicians, and business staff. A very real benefit of offerings from MGMA is that the context of their programs and other resource media is specific to the work environment. The content of most programs and materials from MGMA will be relevant to clinical practice staff and operations.

In addition to face-to-face conferences and seminars, MGMA offerings include technology-based resources such as Webcasts, audio conferences, and online study options. The MGMA menu of training options offers selections to meet most specific requirements for content, access, or cost. The MGMA Website stores an extensive collection of practice-related articles and guidelines available as a member service.

Other Professional Organizations

Most practice staff who hold medical or clinical degrees or professional certifications will be members of professional organizations that provide services to their academic disciplines. Their services may include certification or recognition of specialty training, and most will provide resources to meet their designated continuing-education requirements. Information about educational opportunities through these organizations typically will be available on their Websites, in their print journals, or through direct mailings. This section addresses only two selected professional associations that provide training in information management. As does MGMA, these organizations make their education resources available in various formats, generally via the Internet or other technology-based media.

The Healthcare Information and Management Systems Society (HIMSS), founded in 1961, provides membership services and resources related to information technology management. These resources include education and professional development materials and seminars, print and online publications, and audio conferences. Additional information about HIMSS is available at www.himss.org.

Whereas HIMSS is primarily focused on the management of information technology, the American Health Information Management Association (AHIMA) provides services in support of managing health information and health information workers. These services include resources for professional development and professional practice. This organization was founded in 1928 and is 50,000 members strong. It offers a very large volume of educational resources specific to health information management and provides excellent networking opportunities for members. Additional information about AHIMA is available at www.ahima.org.

MGMA (and the American College of Medical Practice Executives [ACMPE], its certification body), HIMSS, and AHIMA all recognize career and professional development achievements through fellowship programs. Although criteria for board certification and fellowship designation differ among the three organizations, each process involves a rigorous evaluation of sustained academic and professional practice accomplishments over a period of time. Practice executives who pursue fellowship should develop a structured plan and time line to accomplish that goal.

Web-Based Education

Based on open, nonproprietary standards for sending and receiving multimedia communications, the Internet became the dominant global computer network in the early 1990s. Today, the Internet is pervasive in home, business, and education arenas. The World Wide Web, a global hypertext system, has made the Internet more "user-friendly" through communications protocols that make information accessible via a simple hypertext link.

The "dot-com" era spawned an incredible number of virtual businesses, including many education and training companies. Established businesses and academic institutions exploit the Internet's opportunities as well. Judicious evaluation of these opportunities can yield training to meet specific needs while avoiding travel costs and reducing lost work time.

The key point lies in establishing criteria for evaluating training and education options available. These criteria typically would be some variation on the "cost, access, quality" themes. *Cost* comparisons of a given program within an existing training budget are relatively simple. The difficulty here lies in setting the training budget initially!

The convenience of *access* to online training frequently is a strong selling point. However, a Web seminar that occurs during the busiest time of the practice's operating day usually is not a good option. Therefore, time or day availability restrictions may be important criteria. The length of the training program and the number of staff involved likely are relevant factors as well.

By far the most difficult to evaluate prospectively is the *quality* of an educational offering, online or otherwise. Because the actual content is not available for preview, proxy measures must be used for judgment. The most commonly used proxy criteria include the reputation and credibility of the sponsoring organization, the name recognition of the faculty as experts in the field, and recommendations by colleagues. If information about any of these points is unavailable or insufficient, the "fallback" approach is to examine the promotional materials for answers to some key questions, such as:

- Are meaningful learning objectives specified?
- Do the objectives "fit" with the practice's expectations and desires?
- Do the objectives promise the skill level needed, or are they too basic or too advanced?
- Will additional resources, such as print materials or application models, be provided?
- Has the program been approved for continuing-education credit by professional societies?
- Is the cost acceptable compared to other training options?

Academic Institutions

Brick-and-mortar academic institutions still exist, but most have joined the cyber-world and make at least some of their offerings available in electronic formats. Some institutions have specialized in "distance education"' and serve geographically dispersed populations. For the staff member who wants formal academic credit for learning a job skill (such as accounting), or who wants to earn a degree while remaining employed, a distance- or technology-based option may be the best solution.

Information about programs that offer online courses or degrees in health care management is available from the Association of University Programs in Health Administration (www.aupha.org). Information about programs that offer online courses or degrees in health information management is available from AHIMA (www.ahima.org).

Practically speaking, a training and professional development plan, whether for the practice staff or the medical practice executive, most likely will be some combination of all these resource options. Achieving a good balance between supporting desired and needed training for the staff and the cost to the practice in nonproductive time and financial contribution is challenging.

■ Equipment, Software, and Media Options

Most medical practices have in place at least minimal computer and technology resources that can be used to deliver or access education and professional development opportunities. This section presents a brief overview of the most commonly used technologies for on-the-job training and professional development.

Most office workstations now consist of a personal computer (PC) with various peripheral devices attached. The PC likely will have a suite of applications, such as Microsoft® Office®, which includes word processing, spreadsheet, presentation software, and a database. Workstations in a practice may be networked, perhaps with some shared applications housed on a server, or stand-alone with all programs resident on the individual processors. Whatever the configuration, PCs used to access online resources must have adequate processing speed and sufficient memory to manage multimedia files in real time. In addition to basic word processing and related office applications, specific applications must be resident for receiving some types of files. Many of these applications are available as free downloads, such as Java™, RealPlayer™, or Adobe® Acrobat®.

Some education vendors still make training videos available in videocassette (i.e., VHS) format. These videos can be excellent resources because they are easily accessed, can be viewed by many people at once or consecutively, are easily duplicated, and generally are relatively inexpensive. Projection equipment may be readily available in the practice if this medium has been used for patient education. As with video, "older" audio technology, such as cassette tapes, remains in limited use but may still be a viable option for some training applications. The benefits are similar to those stated for VHS, but strictly audio media are quickly becoming obsolete. By far the larger market for audio and video training materials in portable format is that of the CD (compact disk) or DVD (digital video disk). Newer PCs, including notebooks, have CD-DVD drives as standard features. This will eliminate the need for peripheral playback or projection devices unless the CD-DVD material will be viewed by a group of people simultaneously. Ideally, these computer drives should write as well as read CDs and DVDs.

Streaming audio and video over the Internet is becoming a commonly used option in education programs. The caveat for this format is that the speed of the Internet connection is crucial to the quality of the video received. Additional factors that affect viewing quality are the size and resolution of monitors and the available processing memory. Training via streamed video can take place at the workstation, but productive work cannot be carried out simultaneously.

Interactive media, which require the user to input selections or responses that modify how subsequent information is presented, present one of the best media choices for learning applications. This technology applies learning principles such as involvement, feedback, and repetition to engage the user in the learning process. Not surprisingly, this approach is also more expensive than most of the other options because of the cost of development.

◼ Practice Management Issues

Planning for training and professional development for the practice staff has many facets. Managers must be prepared to determine who will receive what training, when and how the training will occur, and what funds will be provided. These decisions are important elements of managing the practice's human resources.

Establishing Practice Priorities and Topics for Training

Building clinical and business skill sets to achieve strategic goals should be the practice's first priority for allocating training and professional development funds. One of the first tasks in the process of establishing professional development plans is to review the practice's strategic plan. The medical practice executive should review the strategic objectives established for the next two to three years, and pay particular attention to any that require specific key personnel skills to be successful. Training and education funds generally are budgeted for an operating cycle, so the manager should pay particular attention to any skill sets required during or immediately following the budget period.

In addition, the manager should ascertain what expert knowledge or advanced skills personnel must possess to perform their jobs under future conditions as the strategy is implemented. This includes determining the level of knowledge and skills that currently exists and identifying gaps that must be corrected with education and training. A good understanding of these facts is pivotal to setting an appropriate training agenda.

Second priorities for education funds for the staff may include training needed to achieve specialty certifications or earn advanced degrees, or other personal education goals that benefit the practice as well as the individual. These choices may be negotiated with individuals as employment benefits during recruitment.

Lower funding priorities are those that are of interest to individual staff members but do not have a direct return to the practice. These funds may be allocated as rewards for performance or for other reasons.

Communicating Options to Staff

Clinical and professional staff often have their own professional development agenda, which may or may not coincide with the practice's strategy. Negotiating performance objectives with individual staff members is an ideal context in which to discuss their personal development plans and their future with the practice. It is important for the medical practice executive to communicate the practice's strategic goals and to discuss how the employees will contribute to achieving those goals. Rationally, the amount of training resources an employee receives should be directly related to the value that accrues to the practice from the employee's enhanced skill set.

Employees should be involved in decisions about changes to their jobs and any resulting commitments for skills development that will be required, including training options, media, and time allocation. However, the medical practice executive is ultimately responsible for establishing a training plan that will result in the desired learning outcomes without exceeding acceptable cost limits or disrupting business operations.

Providing Support for Education

It is a rare medical practice that can provide full financial and time support for all the educational pursuits of its staff. The direct costs of education can be high, and the hidden costs can be equally as high. Certainly, the practice should bear the majority of costs associated with staff development to support strategic goals. Because an enhanced skill set is an asset to the employee as well, sharing education costs may be appropriate in some situations. The extent of support for education should be clearly established and communicated to affected staff.

Some practices allocate financial resources to reimburse staff for tuition, fees, and other expenses associated with earning an academic degree. Although tuition benefits can be an excellent employee recruiting and retention tactic, a formal policy that specifies eligibility guidelines and funding limitations must be in place. Again, these guidelines should be published and communicated to staff.

Scheduling Flexibility

The business and clinical operations of the practice certainly must be protected, but some flexibility in scheduling that allows staff to pursue education and professional development opportunities generally can be accommodated. In some instances when financial support cannot be provided, a time accommodation may be an acceptable, if less desirable, alternative.

Just as with financial agreements, time accommodations for individual staff members should be negotiated, agreed to by both parties, and documented in accordance with policy. Productive employee time is an organization resource, and decisions about depleting that resource should be made with regard for the value returned to the practice. Priorities for time accommodation for staff should follow the same guidelines as for other elements of the professional development plan.

Evaluating Results and Providing Feedback

Professional development and education programs follow the same general control model as all management activities: plan, implement, evaluate, and provide feedback of evaluation findings. Evaluation and feedback are required to improve future planning and implementation. This should not be perceived as a linear activity, and evaluation and feedback should be occurring continuously at key control points.

The professional development plan itself should be reviewed periodically by the medical practice executive to make any adjustments required by changes in personnel or learning needs. The training budget should be monitored and variances analyzed routinely with other budget elements. Most important, however, is the need to evaluate the actual learning outcomes achieved. Unfortunately, this avenue to determining the practical value of the training program is almost never done. If done at all, rarely is a formal approach used to verify that the training dollars spent resulted in developing the desired knowledge and skills.

One simplistic approach that may be useful to "close the circle" with feedback is for the manager to meet with employees following training events and ask them to evaluate the experience on a few key indicators, such as:

- The instructor's expertise in the subject;
- How well the program met the stated objectives;
- The knowledge or skill gained as a return on time investment; and
- The knowledge or skill gained as a return on financial investment.

Over time, patterns of responses may emerge that affect the medical practice executive's future choices of training approaches for education vendors.

For more about staffing, training, and development, refer to the *Body of Knowledge Review, second edition: Human Resource Management* book.

Chapter 5 **Overseeing Database Management and Maintenance**

Managing Databases and Applications

The ultimate purpose of a *database management system (DBMS)* is to transform large volumes of stored data into actionable information. Medical practice management is full of change and shifting priorities, so the value of an information management system clearly is tied to the ease with which information can be accessed, manipulated, and presented to support decision making. A robust DBMS can provide clinicians and administrative staff with the ability to manage, locate, and share needed information with ease and flexibility.

The majority of medical practice data, such as patient records, treatment reports, accounting data, schedules, and appointments, likely are held in some form of database. Some data sets will be in relatively simple "flat files," such as an *Excel* spreadsheet, that are easily updated and manipulated and require minimal management. Other databases, such as *relational databases* comprising multiple tables of data, require more active management. As with most aspects of management, the first step in planning DBMS development is to conduct a needs assessment.

■ Database Development

If the practice currently utilizes a database management system, answers to the following questions should be considered in the planning process. It may be helpful to rank the questions and attach values to assist in later prioritization.

- Is the existing DBMS adequate to support all relevant job tasks?
- Is the DBMS easy to use and efficient?
- If multiple databases are used, are they stored on different computers?
- Can multiple staff access the same database?
- Are staff adequately trained to use the database effectively for all required job functions?
- Is existing hardware adequate to run the database software for efficient transaction speed?
- Is the current DBMS application outdated regarding available vendor upgrades?

If, however, a DBMS is not currently in place, the medical practice executive should answer the following questions about the practice and the way information is managed as a precursor to defining specific planning and development needs. Again, it may be helpful to rank the questions and assign a point value to assist in prioritizing selection criteria at a later point in the process.

- How is such data as patient demographic information, appointments, inventory, accounting, professional contacts, and projects currently stored?
- Is the current method efficient?
- Is it easy to share data among various users in the practice?
- What types of additional data should be stored?
- Who is or will be responsible for maintaining the data?
- How do you want to manipulate and extract information (i.e., retrieve exact entries, sort data, print reports)?
- Who will use the DBMS?

- What tasks will be performed using the data?
- Will several persons need to access the database?
- Will the current network structure support data sharing?
- How many records will be entered into the DBMS?
- How long will records be maintained?
- Will additional computer hardware be required?
- Are funds available for purchasing additional hardware (if necessary) and the DBMS?
- What level of vendor support will be required?
- What will the required vendor support cost?

■ Buy vs. Build

Two key points should be considered when selecting a database management system. First, the basic user tasks to access, query, and manipulate the database should be easy and intuitive. Second, the DBMS should incorporate comprehensive data management tools for data analysis, report management, and other key practice management tasks.

When it comes to purchasing a DBMS, the preferred business option generally is to buy a vendor product and to use customization as a fallback option.[34] An "off-the-shelf product" is more cost-effective and typically will offer a flexible platform for additional development. However, not all vendor products are created equally. It is important to select a DBMS product carefully, applying accepted principles of vendor evaluation and establishing objective selection criteria. In addition to being cost-effective, the DBMS should be scalable so the application can grow with the practice.

Typically, a team of individuals within the organization will be charged with the responsibility to evaluate and recommend a DBMS for purchase. The selection team should include both technical and managerial personnel as well as representative end users. Once selection criteria are identified from the needs assessment, the team will evaluate a selection of DBMS purchase options.

◼ How a Database Works

Databases are used to compare, sort, order, merge, separate, and connect data. Although other simpler file structures exist, the most common form of database used in health care organizations is the relational database. Data are stored in a relational database using multiple two-dimensional tables, very similar to an *Excel* spreadsheet. The file structure creates "relationships" among variables in the database tables so that data from various tables can be extracted through queries to create user-defined reports. In essence, a relational database acts as *data repository*.[35] When used to its maximum capability, a robust data repository and relational DBMS have the potential to eliminate paper storage. A key point of relational databases is that the number of data fields, records, and files stored for each encounter must be specified *a priori* in the design process.

According to Austin and Boxerman,[36] a DBMS uses a data definition language to define and describe the data within the database. A data manipulation language is then used to access, edit, and extract information stored within the database. A DBMS also uses a *data dictionary* to store a detailed description of each variable captured in the database. A database management system such as SQL Server, Access®, DB2, and Oracle will provide the software tools needed to organize data into usable information in a flexible manner.

◼ Types of Data

The ultimate purpose of a DBMS in practice is to transform data into usable information that is then transformed into action. Databases allow definition of data types and data formats for the stored information. Each variable in a database is contained in a *field*. So, for example, a practice manager would be able to store numeric or alphanumeric data and define the data's length or specific value. An example of a field is a patient's last name. Databases store entered data in a *record*. A record is simply a collection of multiple related fields of data, perhaps about a particular patient or inventory item. For example, a patient's demographic information or clinical data from an encounter would be stored as a record. In the database, records are displayed in an electronic form, where field data may be entered, edited, viewed, and deleted.

Several records with the same related fields of information for entries are referred to as a *database table*. The data contained in the database tables can be presented in a formatted, easy-to-read report. A single report could possibly contain data from many different tables and incorporate a complex set of relationships created by the use of multiple links within the database.

For example, a table named "patient" likely will contain fields including patient identifiers and encounter information. The best way to form tables is express relationships between two key variables. A patient may have one or more visits and may be treated by one or more providers during a visit. If the relationships are logical, the next step is to identify attributes associated with patient, provider, and visit. These attributes become fields assigned to the associated table.[37]

◼ Policies and Procedures

The DBMS administrator should work with key clinical and administrative staff to develop policies and procedures to ensure the security and confidentiality of the practice's identifiable health data. Plans, policies, and procedures should be established for the following DBMS issues at a minimum:

- Regular, routine data backup;
- Journal or log for documenting alternations to operational software;
- Formal process for database maintenance by accountable personnel;
- Physical database security;
- User access control and monitoring; and
- Database recovery plan.

■ Personnel Skills

Two types of personnel are required to successfully implement a DBMS in a medical practice setting – the end users, and DBMS administrators or developers. End-user personnel comprise the majority of the facility staff. They must receive training to develop skills needed to create tables, queries, and electronic forms. End users must be able to perform basic database functions, such as establishing queries, retrieving data according to specifications, and generating routine and special reports. Most will need some level of knowledge of the most commonly used database programs such as SQL, Access®, DB2, and Oracle.

DBMS administrators are responsible for the administrative functions associated with the DBMS. These functions include planning, policy formulation, database design, and end-user workflow analysis. DBMS administrators implement the technical details of a DBMS, manage the information data repositories, and apply and monitor the security measures established to protect the stored data. A DBMS administrator must have technical expertise in the design, implementation, and maintenance of a DBMS. As specified by Campbell,[38] the DBMS administrator should have the ability to:

- Interpret data models;
- Develop database structures;
- Program, configure, and maintain relational databases;
- Develop and manipulate complex data sets;
- Provide technical guidance and leadership;
- Install, maintain, modify, and upgrade database software; and
- Implement and troubleshoot programming changes and modifications.

In addition, the DBMS administrator must have robust knowledge of computer and network security systems, applications, procedures, and techniques. Technical-writing skills are desirable as well.

Chapter 6 **Protecting Patient and Practice Data Systems**

◼ Ensuring Network and System Security

The medical practice must ensure that its electronic network and information systems are secure. Any security program in a health care organization should have three principal goals:

1. Protecting the informational privacy of patient-related data;

2. Ensuring the integrity of information; and

3. Ensuring the availability of information to the appropriate individuals in a timely manner.

Broadly, these goals deal with issues of confidentiality, privacy, and security of information. Many persons use these terms interchangeably when dealing with protecting information. Their specific definitions are, however, different. *Confidentiality* refers to the provider's obligation to maintain patient information in a manner that will protect the patient's privacy, and to refrain from allowing other parties to access the information. Patients expect personally identifiable information collected about them to be used solely for the purpose for which it was gathered, and not released by the provider to other parties.

Privacy is the right of an individual to control disclosure of his or her personal information. This means that, with few exceptions, the medical practice cannot release patient information to third parties without the express consent from the patient. Data and information collected by the practice must be shared only with those authorized to have it.

Security refers to the means used to control access and protect information from accidental or intentional disclosure to unauthorized persons, and from being altered, destroyed, or lost. Regarding the patient's expectation that his or her data will be used for its intended purpose, the practice must protect information against theft or improper use. Security should also encompass auditing, educational and awareness programs, and policies.

Health Insurance Portability and Accountability Act

With the enactment in 1996 of HIPAA, a patient's right to have his or her health information kept private and secure became more than just an ethical obligation of physicians and their practices. HIPAA deals with a variety of issues important to the medical practice. A summary of the HIPAA Privacy Rule is available on the U.S. Department of Health and Human Services (HHS) Website (go to www.hhs.gov/ocr, select Health Information Privacy, and then choose Privacy Rule Summary under the General Background Information list).

The HIPAA administrative simplification aspects can be grouped into three major components: (1) electronic transactions; (2) unique identifiers for individuals, employers, health plans, and health care providers; and (3) security and privacy.

The electronic transaction component of administrative simplification is intended to reduce the costs and administrative burdens of health care by making possible the standardized, electronic transmission of certain administrative and financial transactions that were previously carried out manually on paper. The final regulations identified the following administrative functions and require these functions to be performed electronically whenever possible:

- Health care claim or encounter documentation;
- Claim payment and remittance advice;
- Health care claim status;
- Coordination of benefits;
- Eligibility for a health plan;
- Referral certification and authorization;
- Enrollment and disenrollment in a health plan; and
- Premium payments.

With the adoption of standards for electronic transmission, a HIPAA-specified transaction typically requires the use of an *electronic signature*, generally defined as the act of attaching an identifying name or code by electronic means. The electronic signature process involves the authentication of the signer's identity, a signature process according to system and software instructions, binding of the signature to the document, and nonalterability after the signature has been affixed to the document. The HHS proposes that a cryptographically based digital signature be adopted as the standard. The same legal weight is associated with a digital signature as with an original signature on a paper document.

Providers who transmit health information electronically in connection with any of the standard transactions mentioned above are required to obtain a National Provider Identifier (NPI). Implementation of the NPI will eliminate the need for providers to use different identification numbers as they currently do to identify themselves when conducting standard transactions with multiple health plans. As specified in the NPI Final Rule,[39] many health plans, including Medicare, Medicaid, private health insurance issuers, and all health care clearinghouses, must accept and use NPIs in standard transactions by May 23, 2007.

Employers may need to be identified when they transmit information to health plans to enroll or disenroll an employee as a participant. Whenever information about the employer is to be transmitted electronically, it will be beneficial to identify the employer by using a standard identifier. On May 31, 2002, HHS published the Final Rule for Standard Unique Employer Identifiers.[40] This rule requires that the Internal Revenue Service (IRS) Employer Identification Number be used as the standard identifier of employers in HIPAA-covered transactions.

The HIPAA legislation recognized that employing a unique identifier for individuals would be a beneficial component of administrative simplification, by improving quality of care and reducing administrative costs. However, opinion on the specifics of the individual identifier has been deeply divided. HHS has decided to proceed cautiously, given the level of controversy surrounding this issue.

The HIPAA Privacy Rule established standards for who may have access to *protected health information (PHI)* and how the information can be used. Key provisions of these standards include:

- Patients' access to their medical records;
- Notification to patients of their providers' privacy practices;
- Limits on how providers may use personal medical information;
- Restrictions and limits on the use of patient information for marketing purposes; and
- Ensurance that providers take reasonable steps to make their communications with patients confidential.

The Privacy Rule also requires physicians and their practices to establish policies and procedures to protect the confidentiality of PHI about their patients, including a description of staff who have access to protected information, how this information will be used, and when it will be disclosed. The rule also requires physician practices to train their employees regarding their privacy procedures and to designate an individual responsible for ensuring that the procedures are followed.

HIPAA requires health care employees to use or share only "minimum necessary" information to do their jobs effectively. The minimum necessary requirement does not apply, however, to treatment.

Clinical staff can see a patient's entire record and freely share information with other clinicians who care for that patient if necessary.

The Security Rule sets the standards for ensuring that only those who should have access to electronic protected health information will actually have access. The rule requires a three-pronged strategy: technical safeguards, administrative safeguards, and physical safeguards. Technical safeguards include access controls, audit controls, data integrity controls, authentication, and transmission security. Administrative safeguards include backup plans, disaster recovery plans, an emergency-mode operation plan, and testing and revision procedures. Physical safeguards include facility security, device and media control, and workstation use and security.

◼ Accountability

HIPAA identifies data confidentiality, integrity, availability, and accountability as the primary areas of concern. Amatayakul[41] suggests several types of events that can occur in these four areas and recommends the preventive approaches outlined in Exhibit 5.

Access controls are measures to ensure that only authorized personnel have access to a computer or network or to certain applications or data. The most common way to control access is through user identification and strong passwords. Passwords should be at least six characters in length and contain a combination of alpha, numeric, and "special" (e.g., %, $) characters. In addition, passwords should be changed routinely every 30 to 60 days.

To supplement access controls, Johns[42] recommends other automatic security functions to be in place, including the following:

- Automatically terminating a user's session after a predetermined period of inactivity;
- Routinely logging all transactions automatically, including additions, deletions, or changes to the data;
- Automatically and regularly producing and monitoring audit trails;

EXHIBIT 5.
Proactive Tactics to Prevent Adverse Data Events

Adverse Event	Preventive Tactic
Unauthorized access or disclosure to an unauthorized person	The most basic method used to prevent breach of confidentiality due to unauthorized system access is to create different levels of access based on what information individuals need to perform their jobs.
Modification, alteration, or destruction of data resulting in data integrity or data availability problems	Determine which individuals need to modify, alter, or delete data based on job requirements, and grant access to these functions accordingly. Some individuals may need only to view the information and therefore their data access will be in a strictly "read-only" mode.
System attacks that compromise system functionality and data availability	System attacks can occur in a variety of ways, ranging from unauthorized access by hackers to unprotected downloaded files and e-mails containing viruses and worms. A variety of technological solutions, ranging from firewalls to antiviral software, should be in place to rectify these attacks.
Former or disgruntled employees accessing the system and modifying, altering, and/or deleting data	This is probably the greatest risk compromising data integrity, and one of the most difficult to manage proactively. One key approach is to have a procedure in place for removing access rights immediately upon employee termination or when retaliation is anticipated.

- Maintaining current antivirus software on the network and workstation personal computers, and routinely scanning for viruses and worms; and

- Immediately revoking access privileges when an employee leaves the organization or is terminated.

◼ Confidentiality of Information

A major purpose of the HIPAA Privacy Rule is to define and limit the circumstances in which an individual's protected health information may be used or disclosed. As a rule, the medical practice may not use or disclose PHI except:

- As the Privacy Rule permits or requires; or

- As authorized in writing by the individual who is the subject of the information or the individual's personal representative.

It is very important to rely on professional ethics and best judgment, as well as published guidelines, in deciding which permissive uses and disclosures to make regarding patient information. The medical practice is permitted, but not required, to use and disclose PHI without an individual's authorization for the purposes or situations shown in Exhibit 6.

The medical practice must develop and implement policies and procedures for releasing PHI. Procedures also must be established to document the process of restricting access and use of PHI based on employees' specific job roles. These policies and procedures must identify the individuals who need access to PHI to carry out their duties, the categories of PHI to which access is needed, and any conditions under which they need the information to do their jobs.

These policies and procedures should reference state regulations and other federal regulations that govern the disclosure of protected patient information, such as the Confidentiality of Alcohol and Drug Abuse Patient Records Regulation, the Medicare Conditions of Participation, and the Clinical Laboratory Improvement Act, if applicable.

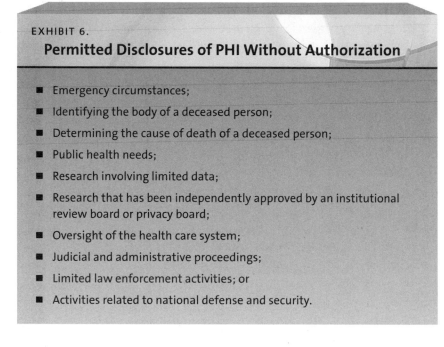

EXHIBIT 6.

Permitted Disclosures of PHI Without Authorization

- Emergency circumstances;
- Identifying the body of a deceased person;
- Determining the cause of death of a deceased person;
- Public health needs;
- Research involving limited data;
- Research that has been independently approved by an institutional review board or privacy board;
- Oversight of the health care system;
- Judicial and administrative proceedings;
- Limited law enforcement activities; or
- Activities related to national defense and security.

System Integrity

System integrity is grounded in protecting the information system and data against tampering. Unauthorized access is regarded as one of the most serious threats to security in any information system. Prevention of unauthorized access relies on a good access control system. Passwords and user identification have been discussed previously as the primary mechanisms for controlling access to the information system and its data by practice staff.

In dealing with unauthorized access to systems over the Internet, the best defense is a *firewall*, special hardware and software that blocks access to computer resources. Firewall software screens the activities of a person who logs on to a Website. The firewall allows retrieval and viewing of certain authorized material but blocks attempts to change the information or to access other resources that reside on the network or computer. The software screens for viruses and for active attempts to invade company resources through open communication lines.

Encryption is another way to limit unauthorized access of confidential information sent over the Web. Encryption scrambles messages at the sending end and descrambles them at the receiving end. Encryption is also used to authenticate the sender or recipient of a message, verifying that the user is indeed the party it claims to be, and to keep messages private.

Maintaining the integrity and accuracy of data, just like maintaining the integrity of the system, relies on good access control. Johns[43] recommends several ways in which the integrity of data can be protected:

- Tight control over authorization to make data modifications;

- Edit and control features to prevent users from making errors; and

- Procedures and techniques to maintain internal consistency of data.

■ Physician and Staff Responsibilities

Formal confidentiality statements must be signed by all practice staff, including physicians, at least annually. These statements should include language indicating that the signer understands and will adhere to the medical practice's policies and procedures to maintain the security of patient information. Recommendations for content in the confidentiality statement[44] include specifying that practice staff will:

- Not use practice e-mail for personal messages;

- Never open or redistribute attached files from an unknown source;

- Never send confidential patient information in an e-mail unless it is encrypted;

- Always verify the address line of an e-mail before it is sent;

- Never share passwords;

- Never log in to the information system with someone else's password;

- Always keep computer screens pointed away from public view; and

- Never remove computer equipment, disks, or software from the facility without the express permission of the practice manager.

Organizations such as the Medical Group Management Association offer policies manuals that cover these and many other protocols:

- Disaster management;

- Stolen or lost computers or access cards; and

- Personal use of practice-owned equipment.

In-service education and training should be conducted annually to reinforce privacy and security issues. In addition, one person, potentially the medical practice executive, should be responsible for monitoring physician and staff confidentiality and security practices.

Consequences for breaching privacy and security practices should be explicitly stated and communicated to all staff. Consequences established by the practice should be determined by the severity of the infraction and may range from written warnings to immediate termination.

In addition to disciplinary action by the medical practice, the staff should understand that a confidentiality or security breach could result in a civil or criminal penalty. The Office for Civil Rights may impose monetary penalties of up to $100 for each requirement or prohibition violated, up to a maximum of $25,000 per year. Criminal penalties apply for certain actions such as knowingly obtaining protected health information in violation of the law. Criminal penalties can range up to $50,000 and up to one year in prison for certain offenses; up to $100,000 and up to five years in prison if the offenses are committed under "false pretenses"; and up to $250,000 and up to ten years in prison if the offenses are committed with the intent to sell, transfer, or use protected health information for commercial advantage, personal gain, or malicious harm.

Conclusion

PLANNING FOR, selecting, implementing, and managing information resources for a medical practice constitute a challenging, dynamic responsibility, albeit one that is critical to the organization's success. The knowledge base changes continually and relatively rapidly. Decisions about information products cannot be made in isolation, as interoperability of information technology is required to support seamless health care for individuals.

No other domain of the medical practice executive's knowledge is "blessed" with the degree of regulation and external oversight that is applied in health information management. The stakes are high; an individual's right to privacy and the assurance of information security are at risk. The accountability for protecting those rights falls to the practice manager.

The savvy medical practice executive will identify reliable sources of information and good advisers with experience in information management. Both types of resources can provide guidance in balancing the need for access to information for business and patient care needs with the need to protect the security and confidentiality of that same information.

Exercises

THESE QUESTIONS have been retired from the ACMPE Essay Exam question bank. Because there are so many ways to handle various situations, there are no "right" answers, and thus no answer key. Use these questions to help you practice responses in different scenarios.

1. As the administrator of a small group practice, you are responsible for maintaining information systems. The practice recently made a significant investment in a new electronic health record (EHR) system. Several physicians have asked you to devise a plan to ensure the security of the EHR system and the confidentiality of patient information.

   Describe the critical elements of the plan.

2. You are the administrator of a 10-physician, single-specialty practice. The practice's existing information system is aging and has very poor vendor support. The physicians have asked you to help them select a replacement system. One prospective vendor convinced one of the physicians at a trade show that the company's product was developed specifically for your specialty. Now several other physicians in the group are excited about features in the system that will help support their patient and medical record management needs.

Describe how you would handle this situation.

3. You are the administrator of a large primary-care medical practice. Lately, numerous patients have complained about busy signals and an inability to reach the practice by telephone.

    Describe how you would evaluate the situation and prescribe a course of action.

4. You are the administrator of a five-physician single-specialty medical group that has made the decision to proceed with installation of an electronic health record (EHR) system. The partnership has selected and executed a contract with the software vendor. Installation and training is to commence within the next 30 days. One of the physician partners has come to you to express concerns about his ability to change from charts to electronic records. He wants to be an exception and remain on paper charts. Another physician partner, excited about the forward momentum of electronic technology, wants you to investigate voice dictation software he has been reading about and have it installed at the same time as the EHR system.

    Describe how would you handle this situation.

5. You are the administrator of a 25-physician internal-
    medicine group with multiple locations. After the imple-
    mentation of a compliance plan, physician documentation
    and dictation increased substantially. The cost of tran-
    scription services has increased 15 percent in the last year
    because of this increased volume. One of the junior part-
    ners recently saw a demonstration of a voice-recognition
    transcription software package and has requested that the
    group buy the software for her use. A number of the other
    physicians are aware of her enthusiasm and are pushing for
    the group to buy the package for them as well. The finance
    committee wants you to present an analysis of the appro-
    priateness of this voice-recognition transcription software.

    Describe how would you handle this situation.

6. You are the administrator of a medical group practice that outsources its transcriptions. You have signed a business associate agreement with the transcription service. A local attorney's office that uses the same transcription service has just notified you that they mistakenly received and opened a batch of your practice's transcriptions.

    Describe how you would handle this situation.

Notes

1. Reprinted from *MGMA Connexion*, May-June 2008, with permission of Medical Group Management Association. All rights reserved.

2. Healthcare WLAN Application Survey Results, 2007. www.arubanetworks.com/pdf/technology/whitepapers/wp_Healthcare_WLAN_trends.pdf (accessed Dec. 7, 2007).

3. K. Terry, "Doctors Are Getting More Tech Savvy," Medical Economics, Aug. 3, 2007. www.memag.com/memag/Health+Information+Technology%3A+E-Prescribing/Doctors-are-getting-more-tech-savvy/ArticleStandard/Article/detail/443729 (accessed Jan. 22, 2008).

4. F. Bazzoli, "Physician IT Adoption 'Pitiful,'" *Healthcare IT News*, Nov. 14, 2007. www.healthcareitnews.com/story.cms?id=8137 (accessed Jan. 22, 2008).

5. J. Agar, *Constant Touch: A Global History of the Mobile Phone* (London: Icon Books, 2003), 19.

6. C. Bechtel, "IT Office Visits," *Journal of AHIMA* 76 no. 8 (2005): 38–40, 42.

7. Ibid.

8. "Clinical Pathways," www.openclinical.org/clinicalpathways.html (accessed Oct. 13, 2005).

9. G. Amori, "Communication with Patients and Other Customers: The Ultimate Loss Control Tool," in *The Risk Management Handbook for Healthcare Organizations*, ed. R. Carroll (San Francisco: Jossey-Bass, 2004), 821.

10. Myron D. Fottler, John D. Blair, J. D. Whitehead, M. D. Luas, and G. T. Savage, "Assessing Key Stakeholders: Who Matters to Hospitals and Why?" *Hospital and Health Services Administration* 34, no. 4 (1989): 527.

11. Ryerson University, "Survey Techniques," www.ryerson.ca/~mjoppe/ResearchProcess (accessed Sept, 20, 2005).

12. American Statistical Society (ASA), "ASA Series: What Is a Survey?" www.amstat.org/sections/srms/brochures (accessed Sept. 20, 2005).

13. Ibid.

14. Ryerson University, "Survey Techniques."

15. Carol Verret, "Creating a Culture of Customer Service," www.hotel-online.com/Trends/CarolVerret (2000; accessed Sept. 20, 2005).

16. Ibid.

17. California State University, Fullerton, "Telephone Etiquette," www.fullerton.edu/it/services (accessed Sept. 18, 2005).

18. Kim Mulvihill, "Bedside Manner," www.sfgate.com/cgi-bin/article.cgi?file= (2001; accessed Sept. 11, 2005).

19. Ibid.

20. J. Glaser, "IT Assessment Demands Measured Approach. HHN Most Wired," www.hhnmostwired.com (accessed Aug. 31, 2005).

21. Matthew Vuletich, "Learning Curve: So You're Going to Purchase an EHR System – Got a Map?" *MGMA e-Connection* no. 79 (June 2005); M. Vuletich, "Learning Curve: Information Technology Infrastructure: Know How to Talk the Talk," *MGMA e-Connexion* no. 82 (August 2005).

22. S. Cohen, "Emerging Benefits of Integrated IT Systems," *Healthcare Executive* 20, no. 5 (2005): 14–18.

23. E. L. May, "The Transformational Power of IT: Experience from Patient Safety Leaders," *Healthcare Executive* 20, no. 5 (2005): 8–13.

24. G. Fajkus and H. Wurtz, "Early Input Makes for Successful System Output: Getting Executives Involved Early for System Implementation Decisions," *MGMA Connexion* 5, no. 5 (2005): 38–43.

25. D. Scalise, "Where the Patient and Technology Meet," *Hospital & Health Networks* 79, no. 8 (2005): 34–42.

26. T. Moore and S. Roberts, "Worlds Collide: A Look at Wireless Systems Convergence in Health Care Facilities," *Health Facilities Management* 18, no. 8 (2005): 31–34.

27. C. Pope, "The Hereafter: Why IT Security Matters to Your Practice Even After the HIPAA Security Rule Deadline," *MGMA Connexion* 5, no. 6 (2005): 36–41.

28. Ibid.

29. M. K. Amatayakul, *Electronic Health Records: A Practical Guide for Professionals and Organizations,* 2nd ed. (Chicago: American Health Information Management Association, 2004).

30. Healthcare Financial Management Association, *Dotting the i's and Crossing the t's: Ensuring the Best IT Contract,* promotional material (2004).

31. D. J. Slovensky and P. E. Paustian, "Training the Adult Learner in Health Care Organizations," in *Guide to Effective Staff Development in Health Care Organizations: A Systems Approach to Successful Training,* ed. Patrice Spath (San Francisco: Jossey-Bass, 2002), 99–112.

32. B. I. Mygrant and M. C. McMann, "Selecting Appropriate Training Methods," in *Guide to Effective Staff Development in Health Care Organizations: A Systems Approach to Successful Training,* ed. Patrice Spath (San Francisco: Jossey-Bass, 2002), 79–97.

33. R. J. Wager and R. Weigand, "Measuring the Organizational Impact of Training Programs," in *Guide to Effective Staff Development in Health Care Organizations: A Systems Approach to Successful Training,* ed. Patrice Spath (San Francisco: Jossey-Bass, 2002), 113–125.

34. D. T. Jones, R. Duncan, L. Michael, M. L. Langberg, and M. M. Shabot, "Technology Architecture Guidelines for a Health Care System," *Proceedings of the 2000 AMIA Symposium* (2002), 399–402.

35. R. J. Campbell, "Database Design: What HIM Professionals Need to Know," *Perspectives in Health Information Management* 1 (2004). http://library.ahima.org/xpedio/groups/public/documents/ahima/pub_bok1_024637.html.

36. C. J. Austin and S. Boxerman, *Information Systems for Healthcare Management,* 6th ed. (Foundation of the American College of Healthcare Executives, 2003).

37. D. T. Mon, "Relational Database Management: What You Need to Know," *Journal of AHIMA* 74, no. 10 (2003): 40–45.

38. Campbell, "Database Design."

39. Department of Health and Human Services, 45 CFR Part 162, HIPAA Administrative Simplification: Standard Unique Health Identifier for Health Care Providers; Final Rule, *Federal Register* (Jan. 23, 2004), 3433–3469.

40. Department of Health and Human Services, 45 CFR Part 162, HIPAA Administrative Simplification: Standard Unique Health Identifier for Health Care Providers; Final Rule, *Federal Register* (May 31, 2002), 3433–3469.

41. Amatayakul, *Electronic Health Records.*

42. M. L. Johns, *Information Management for Health Professions,* 2nd ed. (Albany, NY: Delmar, Thomson Learning, 2002).

43. Ibid.

44. hcPRO. *Preserving Privacy and Security: HIPAA Training Handbook for Healthcare Organizations* (Marblehead, MA: The Healthcare Compliance Company, 2004).

Glossary

confidentiality – The protection of individually identifiable information from access by nonauthorized parties.

data dictionary – Compilation of detailed descriptions of each variable captured in a specified database.

data repository – A "warehouse" of data elements, captured from multiple points of entry; data may be accessed by authorized users even if they did not perform the data capture; prevents redundant data capture and storage.

database management system (DBMS) – A database system that transforms large volumes of stored data into actionable information.

database table – Several records with the same related fields of information for individual entries.

databases – Information storehouses used to compare, sort, order, merge, separate, and connect data.

electronic signature – Authentication of a document or file using an electronic unique identifier, ideally one that is encrypted.

encryption – A way to limit unauthorized access of confidential information sent over the Web. Encryption scrambles messages at the sending end and descrambles them at the receiving end.

external stakeholder – Individuals and organizations that funcion outside of the organization, such as vendors, patients, and other physician practices.

field – A data element or variable captured electronically; for example, a patient's date of birth.

firewall – Special hardware and software that blocks access to computer resources.

handheld device – Portable computer hardware that allows data capture and access at the point-of-care (e.g., personal digital assistant).

Health Insurance Portability and Accountability Act of 1996 (HIPAA) – Health care legislation that affects health providers in myriad ways; the legislation specifically addresses storage, dissemination, and access to protected health information.

interface stakeholder – Individuals who function both internally and externally, such as hospital medical staff.

internal stakeholder – Any individual who works wholly within the organization, such as office staff.

monitoring devices – Biomedical instruments that capture measurements electronically, eliminating the need for manual entry or transfer of data.

parking lot – A meeting-management technique where items unrelated to the agenda are recorded separately for later attention.

portals – Filters that allow only authorized users to gain entry to information systems.

privacy – The right of an individual to maintain control over his or her personal information.

project management systems – Integrated management and planning tools that help manage an implementation process.

protected health information (PHI) – Individually identifiable health information; as defined by the Health Insurance Portability and Accountability Act, this includes all information (including demographics) related to a person's physical or mental health condition, provision of care, and payment for care.

record – A collection of multiple data fields in an electronic storage medium.

relational database – A database that uses two-dimensional tables to create relationships among variables in the database tables.

request for information (RFI) – The first contact with potential vendor for an information system product; used to gather basic information for comparing several products.

request for proposal (RFP) – The formal process for achieving a vendor's bid for an information system solution.

security – Physical and electronic methods to control access and protect information from nonauthorized access, alteration, or destruction.

servers – Hardware components, similar to those in normal personal computers, that provide the "brains" of the information systems.

telehealth – A system using two-way links between the physician's office and either the patient's home or business location for the purpose of consultations; designed to cut costs of time and travel included in traditional consultations.

workstations – Interface points between the human care providers and support personnel and the information technology systems that assist in providing quality care to patients.

Bibliography

Amatayakul, M. K. *Electronic Health Records: A Practical Guide for Professionals and Organizations,* 2nd ed. (Chicago: American Health Information Management Association, 2004).

American Health Information Management Association. *HIPAA in Practice: The Health Information Manager's Perspective.* (Chicago: American Health Information Management Association, 2004).

American Health Information Management Association. "Practice Brief: Writing an Effective Request for Proposal (RFP)." *Journal of the American Health Information Management Association* 69, no. 7 (1998).

Austin, C. J., & S. Boxerman. *Information Systems for Healthcare Management,* 6th ed. (Chicago: Foundation of the American College of Healthcare Executives, 2003).

Baron, R. J., E. L. Fabens, M. Schiffman, & E. Wolf. "Electronic Health Records: Just Around the Corner? Or over the Cliff?" *Annals of Internal Medicine* 143, no. 3 (2005): 222–226.

Bechtel, C. "IT Office Visits." *Journal of AHIMA* 76, no. 8 (2005): 38–40, 42.

Bureau of Primary Health Care. "Request for Proposals (RFP) for an Automated Clinical Practice Management System [Sample]. bphc.hrsa.gov/chc/SIMIS/PIS/ PIS_RFP.asp (accessed April 2004).

Campbell, R. J. "Database Design: What HIM Professionals Need to Know." *Perspectives in Health Information Management* 1, no. 6 (2004). Also available at library. ahima.org/xpedio/groups/ public/documents/ahima/pub_bok1_024637.html.

———. "What the Health Care Administrator Needs to Consider When Purchasing Personal Computers." *Health Care Manager* 22, no. 1 (2003): 21–26.

Centers for Medicare and Medicaid Services. "HIPAA 101: The Basics of Administrative Simplification." www.cms.hhs.gov/ hipaa/hipaa2.

————. "HIPAA Electronic Transactions and Code Set Compliance Materials."
www.cms.hhs.gov/hipaa/hipaa2.

————. HIPAA Information Series for Providers. www.cms.hhs.gov/hipaa/
hipaa2.

————. HIPAA Security Educational Paper Series. www.cms.hhs.gov/hipaa/
hipaa2.

————. "Provider HIPAA Readiness Checklist." www.cms.hhs.gov/hipaa/hipaa2.

Cohen, S. "Emerging Benefits of Integrated IT Systems." *Healthcare Executive*
20, no. 5 (2005): 14–18.

Fajkus, G., & H. Wurtz. "Early Input Makes for Successful System Output: Getting Executives Involved Early for System Implementation Decisions."
MGMA Connexion 5, no. 5 (2005): 38–43.

Glaser, J. "IT Assessment Demands Measured Approach. HHN Most Wired."
www.hhnmostwired.com (retrieved Aug. 31, 2005).

Haugh, R. "Wiring Docs." Hospitals and Health Networks 78, no. 11 (2004):
4–46, 55.

hcPRO. *Preserving Privacy and Security: HIPAA Training Handbook for Healthcare
Organizations.* (Marblehead, MA: The Healthcare Compliance Company,
2004).

Healthcare Financial Management Association. Dotting the i's and Crossing
the t's: Ensuring the Best IT Contract. Promotional material (2004).

Johns, M. L. Information Management for Health Professions, 2nd ed. (Albany, NY: Delmar, Thomson Learning, 2002).

Jones, D. T., R. Duncan, M. L. Langberg, & M. M. Shabot. "Technology Architecture Guidelines for a Health Care System." Proceedings of the 2000
AMIA Symposium (2000), 399–402.

Kiel, J. M., & R. J. Campbell. "Designingyourpractice.com: Ten Steps to an
Informative Website." MDComputing (November/December 1999):
30–33.

Kuyper, L., & C. Shanks. "Two Viewpoints: The Preparation of a Request for
Proposal." *Journal of the American Health Information Management Association* 59, no. 7 (1988): 23–27.

May, E. L. "The Transformational Power of IT: Experience from Patient Safety
Leaders." *Healthcare Executive* 20, no. 5 (2005): 8–13.

McWay, D. *Legal Aspects of Health Information Management,* 2nd ed. (Clinton
Park, NY: Delmar, Thomson Learning, 2003).

Migliore, S. "Information Technology in the Medical Practice." *Physician's News Digest.* www.physiciansnews.com/computers/903.migliore.html.

Miller, C. "Process, Priorities, and the Strategic Plan: How to Request New Information Technology." *Journal of the American Health Information Management Association* 74, no. 8 (2003): 42–46, 48.

Mon, D. T. "Relational Database Management: What You Need to Know." *Journal of AHIMA* 74, no. 10 (2003): 40–45.

Moore, T., & S. Roberts. "Worlds Collide: A Look at Wireless Systems Convergence in Health Care Facilities." *Health Facilities Management* 18, no. 8 (2005): 31–34.

Mygrant, B. I., & M. C. McMann. "Selecting Appropriate Training Methods," in *Guide to Effective Staff Development in Health Care Organizations: A Systems Approach to Successful Training.* Patrice Spath, ed. (San Francisco: Jossey-Bass, 2002), 79–97.

Oz, E. *Management Information Systems,* 4th ed. (Boston: Course Technology, Thomson Learning, 2004).

Pope, C. "The Hereafter: Why IT Security Matters to Your Practice Even After the HIPAA Security Rule Deadline." *MGMA Connexion* 5, no. 6 (2005): 36–41.

Scalise, D. "Where the Patient and Technology Meet." *Hospital & Health Networks* 79, no. 8 (2005): 34–42.

Slovensky, D. J., & P. E. Paustian. "Training the Adult Learner in Health Care Organizations," in *Guide to Effective Staff Development in Health Care Organizations: A Systems Approach to Successful Training.* Patrice Spath, ed. (San Francisco: Jossey-Bass, 2002), 99–112.

U.S. Department of Health and Human Services. "Fact Sheet: Protecting the Privacy of Patient's Health Information." (April 14, 2003).

Vuletich, M. "Learning Curve. Information Technology Infrastructure: Know How to Talk the Talk." *MGMA e-Connexion* no. 82 (August 2005).

———. "Learning Curve: So You're Going to Purchase an EHR System – Got a Map?" *MGMA e-Connexion* no. 79 (June 2005).

Wager, R. J., & R. Weigand. "Measuring the Organizational Impact of Training Programs," in *Guide to Effective Staff Development in Health Care Organizations: A Systems Approach to Successful Training.* Patrice Spath, ed. (San Francisco: Jossey-Bass, 2002), 113–125.

Index

Note: (ex.) indicates exhibit.